When It Happens to You

A Practical Guide Through Breast Cancer

EARLENE DAL POZZO, M.D.

AND

JOANN DILTS, M.A.

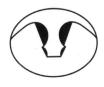

Bull Publishing Company

Bull Publishing Company
P.O. Box 208
Palo Alto, CA 94302-0208
Phone (650) 322-2855
Fax (650) 327-3300
www.bullpub.com

Distributed in the United States by:
Publishers Group West
1700 Fourth Street
Berkeley, CA 94710

Publisher: James Bull
Production: Publication Services, Inc.
Cover Design: Robb Pawlak, Pawlak Design
Cover Art: Mary Bonnell
Interior Design: Publication Services, Inc.
Printer: Malloy Lithographing, Inc.

Dal Pozzo, Earlene, date-
    When it happens to you: a practical guide through breast
cancer / Earlene Dal Pozzo & Joann Dilts.
        p. cm.
    Includes bibliographical references and index.
    ISBN 0-923521-49-6
    1. Breast–Cancer–Popular works. I. Dilts, Joann, date- II. Title.

RC280.B8 D34 2000
616.99'449–dc21   99-087055

Contents

Preface

There are many books about breast cancer and about cancer in general. Fat, complicated technical books talk about the medical facts, which can be confusing and frightening. Others are more personal—they relate individual experiences, they contain the poetry and art that pour from people. Still others provide psychological approaches to dealing with cancer.

In this book we give you some practical suggestions to help make undergoing treatment for breast cancer easier. We will help you create a self-care plan so you can have a sense of autonomy and control in a situation where you may feel you have neither of these things. It is easy to let yourself feel powerless, attacked, and invaded during treatment for cancer. However, when you know how to help yourself, it becomes easier to keep control. Also, by understanding what your disease is, how it will be treated, and how you can participate in many aspects of the healing process, you can overcome some of these feelings.

Just when you want simply to be taken care of, you find yourself faced with having to learn about your disease, having to help your family and friends, having to make decisions about treatment, and having to make sometimes drastic changes in your life to accommodate this disease.

We are breast cancer survivors. Although there were five years between our diagnoses and our treatments were different, many similarities became apparent as soon as we began to talk together. Most striking was that even though we were both from medical families, occasionally we found that we had to struggle to keep control of our treatments. We asked ourselves what it must be like for women and their families who are unfamiliar with the ins and outs of the medical system or for women who lack the extensive support we are fortunate to have. We knew the answer was that it has to be even more difficult for them.

Also, we both had to work out our own ways of coping with our illnesses, and it occurred to us that if others could use what we had learned, they might not need to struggle quite as hard as we did. We hope that from our experiences you will learn something about how to help yourself and how to let others help you so your treatment will be as easy as possible. This is the book we wish we'd had. — **EDP, JD**

Acknowledgments

We are indebted to the many people who were supportive of our efforts: Thanks to Sally and Ted Barrett-Page, Sally Foster, Jill Miller, Terri O'Hara, Shelly Parlente, and Peggy Stall for contributing to and reading sections of the manuscript. Also we want to extend special thanks to Mary Bonnell for her cover art and to Jennifer Caskey, M.D. for her valuable suggestions.

To Don and Paul Daniel with love.

*For my mother, Roberta, who survived before me,
for Steve, Jr. and John, and especially for Steve—
all of you gave me the strength to fight.*

From both of us, our gratitude to Dr. Jennifer Caskey.

chapter 1

Hearing the Diagnosis

No matter how prepared you think you are to hear the news, being told you have breast cancer is simply devastating. Like the assassination of John Kennedy or the explosion of the space shuttle *Challenger,* this is an event you will likely always remember. It is hard to know what to do first, and you may feel terribly alone and confused.

It happens in as many different ways as there are people—a deformity spotted in the mirror, a suspicious mammogram, a lump felt by a lover's hand—and there you are, facing uncertainties you thought happened only to somebody else. There is, however, a big picture, and if you know what it is, you will be better equipped to handle the inevitable problems.

We will try to give you an overview of the process, but there are many different ways of approaching the diagnosis and treatment of breast cancer (see Figure 1.1). If you are uneasy about a lump anywhere, the first thing to do is to see your doctor—this may be your gynecologist or your primary care doctor. You need one of them to help you arrange tests, such as a mammogram, an ultrasound, and/or a biopsy. There are different types of breast cancer, and the specific diagnosis is based on the type of cell from which the cancer originates. It is therefore

1

Discovery and Diagnosis Algorithm

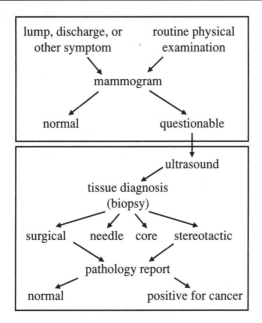

Figure 1.1   *After a normal mammogram or pathology report, a patient may want to discuss with her physician the possibility of preventive treatment for breast cancer using tamoxifen.*

obvious that your doctor needs to get a look at the cells in the lump or thickening or from the area of abnormal findings on a mammogram. No one can diagnose breast cancer for sure by feeling a lump or by looking at findings on a mammogram. In order to make or rule out that diagnosis, a biopsy must be performed.

There are several kinds of biopsies, because there are different ways of getting at the cells: They can be obtained by open, or surgical, biopsy; by fine needle aspiration; or by core needle biopsy. Your gynecologist or primary care physician should refer you to a surgeon who will perform either a surgical or a fine needle biopsy or, alternatively, to a radiologist. In some medical centers, radiologists perform core needle biopsies, which use ultrasound images or stereotactic (computerized) images from the mammogram to help place the needle. Whatever kind of biopsy you have, you will receive some kind of anesthesia, either local or intravenous, and you will probably be awake during this procedure. Having a biopsy is stressful and can be uncomfortable during and afterward—don't plan to go back to work the same day you have had one unless you absolutely have to. If you are given a tranquilizer, you shouldn't drive, and you need to arrange to have someone with you.

The cells from the biopsy are sent to a pathologist, who carefully analyzes samples of the breast tissue and reports the nature and cause of the disease to the surgeon or the radiologist. The surgeon or radiologist then communicates these findings to you and to your primary care physician. It usually takes no more than two or three days to get the results, but the waiting can seem interminable. If the pathology analysis shows that you do indeed have breast cancer, the pathologist will identify the cell type—that is, the kind of cell that went wrong and gave rise to the cancer. The two kinds of cells that most commonly undergo malignant, or cancerous, changes are the duct cells, which carry the secretions of the breast, and the lobular cells, which can produce milk. The majority (86 percent, according to Dr. Susan Love) of cancers begin in the duct cells and 12 percent begin in the lobular cells—the remaining 2 percent arise in other kinds of tissue in the breast.

Once pathologists have identified the cell type, they will then make a determination about whether the cancer cells are confined to the original duct or lobule (in situ) or whether they have spread to surrounding breast tissue (invasive). If the cells have not spread, the name of the cancer might be *ductal carcinoma in situ* or *lobular carcinoma in situ.* If the cells have invaded surrounding tissue, the name of the cancer could be either *invasive (or infiltrating) ductal carcinoma* or *invasive (or infiltrating) lobular carcinoma.* The pathologist will also attribute a nuclear grade to the cells, whether they are ductal or lobular cells. The grade of the tumor is related to the degree of aggressiveness of the cells. Rapidly dividing cells tend to be more aggressive. Tumors are graded 1 through 3 or 4; the higher the number, the more aggressive.

Whatever kind of cancer you have, you will have to make many choices. If the cancer has spread beyond the lymph nodes to other parts of the body, it is called metastatic. Take someone with you when you expect to hear the diagnosis, or if you talk with the doctor on the phone, have a helpful person on an extension or available to talk with the doctor too. Take notes or record the conversation. You may not be able to take in what the doctors are saying or to remember it very well later. Your doctor will probably want to give you the name and phone numbers of yet more doctors.

Regardless of whether the cancer is in situ or invasive, you will need treatment, and here is where the treatment paths begin to diverge (see Figure 1.2). The usual treatment ingredients include surgery, radiation therapy, chemotherapy, and/or hormone therapy; it is which treatment to use and when that become the questions. For invasive cancers, a frequent next step is surgery, either lumpectomy or mastectomy; both of these usually (but not always) include lymph node dissection, especially of those nodes located in the armpit (see Figure 1.3). The goal of surgical treatment is to remove all of the tumor and to try to determine if the cancer has already spread into the lymph nodes, the first place it tends to spread outside the breast.

There are different diagnostic and treatment plans, and they should be designed for your unique situation. The best person to help you make treatment decisions is a medical oncologist. Patients frequently do not see an oncologist until after they have had surgery, but we think you should ask to see an oncologist as soon as you can, because this specialist can evaluate the whole treatment picture for you. Although your surgeon can help you decide which surgery is best and, in fact, may be the person most available to you at this point, you should get as much information as you can before you have surgery. Make an appointment with an

Treatment and Follow-up Algorithm

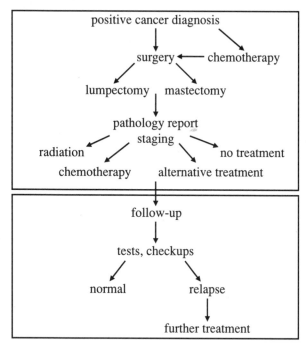

Figure 1.2

oncologist right away **even if you think you may not need chemotherapy or the surgeon says you don't need to right now.** In some cases, the oncologist may recommend chemotherapy even before surgery in an effort to shrink the tumor and kill off cells that may have spread. The surgeon will be able to give you names of oncologists to talk to. If you don't feel you can have a good relationship with the first oncologist you see, ask your primary care doctor or your surgeon for other names so you find someone you trust to guide you through the treatment maze. In summary, the doctors you will see will probably include your primary care physician, a surgeon, or a radiologist, or all three, a medical oncologist, and a radiation oncologist.

Breast Lymph Node Anatomy

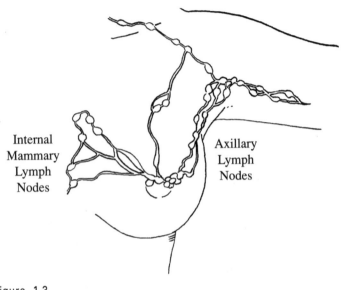

Internal Mammary Lymph Nodes

Axillary Lymph Nodes

Figure 1.3

Your surgeon and your oncologist, if you have one at this point, can help you decide which surgery is best for you. If you choose to have a mastectomy, the surgery may or may not be followed by radiation and/or chemotherapy. Lumpectomy is virtually always followed by radiation therapy to the involved breast to eradicate any possible cancer cells left behind and may also be followed with chemotherapy, especially if there are cancer cells in the lymph nodes.

If any cancer cells are found in the lymph nodes, your doctors will probably want to know if the cancer cells have spread to more distant parts of the body such as the liver, bones, or lungs. When this happens, the cancer is said to have metastasized. Even if there is little suspicion of metastases, you can expect to have a chest X-ray and blood samples taken to evaluate liver functions as part of your initial evaluation. You may also have a bone scan. These tests are in addition to the careful physical examination that you can expect from your surgeon and oncologist.

The information obtained from the biopsy and lymph node dissection is used to decide the stage of your cancer. Staging partly depends on tumor size and whether the cancer cells have spread to any other part of the body. This helps your doctors make treatment recommendations (see Table 1.1).

Okay, these are the possibilities, and we know they sound horrible. The gut reaction to the therapies for cancer is often as devastating as the reaction to the diagnosis itself. All we can say is that there will be rough times, but these treatments can literally be LIFE SAVERS, and the sooner you can view your treatment as your ally, the better things will go. Neither of us was able to accomplish this emotional task very quickly—we are talking months and years—but this is an important thing to try to do. Some people who have been through this recommend hunting around for the treatment and/or physicians that seem right for you—you do have time, and you have to feel confident in the treatment and physicians you choose. We both knew we had highly skilled, caring doctors, so we did not seek second opinions, which might have muddied the waters for us. Plus, we wanted to be on an operating room schedule *yesterday!* However, had we been uneasy about our care, we would have gotten that second opinion. Good doctors are not insulted or hurt if you need another opinion to put your mind at ease.

So, the doctors will give you medical treatment options, and from the very beginning **you need to start designing your own personal treatment plan including augmenting therapies.** These "therapies" may (and we think should) include relaxation, meditation, massage, and exercise. This allows you to transform yourself from a passive victim to an active participant in your treatment. You cannot control the course of your illness, but within limitations you can control much of every day. Like everyone, when we faced this diagnosis, we experienced fear and anxiety—even terror. Using the alternative therapies in our

Table 1.1

Breast Cancer Staging

STAGE 0	■ This is very early breast cancer. Lobular carcinoma in situ (LCIS), ductal carcinoma in situ (DCIS), and breast cancer in situ are other names for this stage of cancer. Stage 0 cancer has not spread within the breast, to the lymph nodes, or to any other part of the body.
STAGE I	■ Breast cancer at this stage is no larger than 2 centimeters (slightly less than an inch) in diameter and also has not spread to the lymph nodes or any other part of the body.
STAGE II	■ The tumor is no larger than 2 centimeters, but has spread to the lymph nodes under the arm. ■ The tumor is 2 to 5 centimeters in diameter and may or may not have spread to the lymph nodes under the arm. ■ The tumor is larger than 5 centimeters, but has not spread to the lymph nodes under the arm.
STAGE IIIA	■ The tumor is smaller than 5 centimeters but has spread to the lymph nodes under the arm. ■ The tumor is larger than 5 centimeters in diameter and has spread to the lymph nodes under the arm.
STAGE IIIB	■ Cancer is found in tissues near the breast such as skin, ribs, or muscles in the chest. ■ Cancer is found in the lymph nodes inside the chest along the sternum (breast bone).
STAGE IV	■ The cancer has spread to the skin and lymph nodes near the collarbone or has spread to other parts of the body. The bone, lungs, liver, or the brain are the most frequent sites of spread.

personal treatment plans increased our sense of well-being while we underwent medical treatments.

Like everyone, we experienced a grieving process similar to that precipitated by the loss of a loved one that was described by Elisabeth Kübler-Ross in 1969. We felt shock, denial, and disbelief; anger; acceptance; and even hope. Sometimes these feelings coexisted in ways useful and not so useful. Finally we began to integrate being a cancer survivor into our lives.

Usually shock and denial doesn't last very long—it can be a few moments to a few hours—because your doctors let you know the facts, and they begin offering you treatment options. They can be pretty persistent in not letting you refuse to face the reality of your disease. If you have been told you have cancer and are reading this book, you probably have already acknowledged the diagnosis. Short-term denial can be helpful because it is one mechanism for keeping your balance as you survive the time periods between tests. Once you have a diagnosis, denial can still be a way of getting an emotional break, but it can harm by interfering with appropriate treatment.

Anger is more enduring. An important useful purpose it can serve is to help you call up your fighting abilities. Anger is the emotion that helps you raise your fist and shout, "This will never get me!!" Anger can be the sustaining force when things get bad; it can help you say, "I have to get through this, and now!" It can help you confront treatment providers who are not doing what you want. Anger, however, can cause you to lash out at those who are trying to help you—your family, friends, and doctors—when what is happening to you is not their fault. Some forms of anger may last for a long time. It helps to recognize anger so you can use it when it is helping you and try to give it up when it is not.

Hope is the positive expectation of staying connected with your life. It offers strength and is the response to wanting to give up. Even in dark times we were able to maintain the belief that we could overcome this ordeal.

Acceptance is the basis for healing. By acceptance we do not mean passive submission to your fate. Rather, positive acceptance of facts combined with a determination to use all your resources to help you heal can be your best ally. It allows you to take charge of what happens, to rearrange your life, to reassess your spiritual values, and to have faith in whatever treatments you choose.

Integration incorporates acceptance. It is how we come to accept that being a breast cancer survivor is part of who we are—but only a part. It is about getting on with living.

First Steps

It is not too soon to be thinking about what reinforces hope and brings comfort. Later on we will help you get started in designing your own personal treatment plan—that is, what you can do for yourself or get others to do for you. Right now you need emotional support, so the first thing to do is to figure out where you're going to get it.

1. *Spouse or Significant Other:* Since your main source of support is probably right at home, it is important to make that person an equal part of what's happening. Cancer happens to families, not just to the affected person. Any significant other needs to be involved with decisions about treatment, choosing physicians, and so on. It is easy for a cancer patient to convince herself that she can do it alone, her partner won't be able to "take it" or is too busy, or she feels guilty about causing trouble, so the significant other gets left out in all the flurry. It's up to patients, with their doctors' help if necessary, to make sure significant others come to appointments and treatments so they understand, and are not left out of, the process. If you live alone, extended family, friends, and organized support groups can provide the essential help you will need.

2. *Friends:* Even if you have a supportive home environment, friends can be a terrific sounding board and support, too. If you live alone or your significant other cannot give you the support you need, friends become even more important, and you should find those who are available to help you with the day-to-day demands of this illness and treatment.

3. Physicians: If you are involved in some kind of health maintenance organization (HMO), you already have a primary care physician. Talk first to that person about who is going to coordinate your care. You will be seeing many different health-care providers, from lab technicians to surgeons, and you need someone to keep them all informed about aspects of your care that are not in their immediate domain. We believe that person should be a medical oncologist. In the very beginning, neither of us had a primary care physician, so we went from one specialist to the next until we were under the wing of our oncologist. It can be overwhelming when you've been sent to one physician, only to be told by that physician you will need to see others.

4. Information About Your Disease: If you are informed about your disease and how it is treated, you'll be able to make better decisions. You should always know what options you have. Ask about the availability of education groups for you and your family. The National Cancer Institute's publications may be available in your doctor's office. They contain straightforward, easy-to-understand information about the medical aspects of cancer. If your doctor hasn't given you these, call the National Cancer Institute at 1-800-4-CANCER or write to the National Cancer Institute, Building 31 Room 10A24, Bethesda, MD 20892 for their free series *What You Need To Know About Cancer.* Ask for the booklet about breast cancer (P017). When you know what sort of treatment you may be having, you can request further booklets about radiation, chemotherapy, anticancer drugs, nutrition, and other subjects.

5. Someone Who's Been There: Find, either through your local cancer society or by word of mouth, someone you can talk to about what it's like to have this disease. (It is really important, we think, that this person be doing well.) Keep in mind your situation will be different in some or many ways from hers, but she still knows how it feels. Also remember that treatment outcomes do not depend on treatment being just like hers; if she is a long-term survivor, that does not mean you have to do exactly what she did or that you should be treated exactly like she was. She can still sympathize with your dislike of sterile atmospheres and two-piece paper gowns, and she can tell you what she learned from her experience.

6. Support Groups: In addition to relying on her friends and family, Earlene went to a six-week support group offered by the hospital where she received her surgery and radiation. Joann stuck to her friends and family for support. Both of us feel fine about our choices. There is a lot of evidence that support groups can be helpful to patients dealing with a breast cancer diagnosis. Dr. David Spiegel at Stanford University demonstrated in 1989 that women with metastatic breast cancer survived longer when they were involved in group psychotherapy. His book, *Living Beyond Limits,* describes some of the other benefits support groups provide for patients with any stage of breast cancer. These include decreasing anxiety and depression, increasing coping skills, and enhancing the ability to confront honestly the challenges that are sure to come. A recent study by V. S. Hegelson and others indicates that support groups for women with early breast cancer that focus on education and strategies for managing the illness and problems associated with treatments increased self-esteem, improved body image, decreased uncertainty about their illness, and enhanced ability to discuss their illness with family and friends.

If you want to give a support group a try, ask your oncologist, radiation oncologist, hospital social worker, or cancer nurse about the availability of support groups. They should be able to recommend a group appropriate for your needs. Sometimes there is a small fee, and sometimes groups are offered at no charge. You can consider reputable groups that offer information about exercise, relaxation techniques, self-hypnosis, meditation, treatment issues, communication techniques, and sexual issues in cancer treatment as well as groups that will support you emotionally. If you try a group and you don't feel comfortable, you may need to find a different one. However, take the time to speak individually with the group leader about your concerns, because she may be able to help.

If you are a minority person, whether African-American, lesbian, Hispanic, or other, and would feel more comfortable in a group made up of or led by members of your own group, there are likely to be services available in large metropolitan areas. If such groups are available, you may need to find them through your own network. Call any of the nationwide organizations that offer cancer services and ask about your own special needs.

There are also support groups for significant others and family members. Finding them may take a little more detective work; a place to start could be the Y-ME hotline (1-800-221-2141).

7. Your Spiritual Counselor: Many people find religious or spiritual groups, rabbis, priests, or ministers to be a source of enormous support during this time. Call to find out what kinds of help they offer. Many offer outreach programs and have someone who will visit you if you let them know you'd like that. If you prefer not to have them come to the hospital, you need to tell them.

Resources

Some resources were helpful to us. These included books, audiocassette tapes (or CDs), pamphlets, and information from national cancer organizations. We recommend getting books from your local library or from your hospital's cancer support department. Then, if you want to buy any, do it. Some cassette tapes may be available only at "new age" stores—don't let that scare you off—and others may be found where ordinary audiotapes are sold. Our resource list at the end of the book will provide names and telephone numbers to get you started.

❏   ❏   ❏

Earlene's Story

The day after I found a pea-sized lump in my breast I went for a mammogram. After a mammogram and ultrasound and a lot of concerned looks from the technician, the radiologist came into the small room where I was lying and, as gently as he could, told me he thought I had malignancies in both breasts. I had not gone for a mammogram to hear this. Thank goodness it turned out to be only in one breast instead of both. I had no risk factors (80% of women diagnosed with breast cancer have no risk factors), my mammograms had always been normal, and, besides, cancer is what happens to other people. Speechless, I nodded and took the name of a surgeon. I was so overwhelmed that I am surprised I didn't put my clothes on backwards. At the same time I was saying to myself, "He's not a pathologist—he can't tell me I have breast cancer." But I knew he wouldn't be saying this unless he was pretty sure. Anyway, it wasn't long before I started crying—the tears came in big waves for weeks and weeks.

That evening I phoned a colleague whose wife I knew had had breast cancer. Could my husband, who went with me everywhere, and I come talk with them? "Sure," they said. I remember that summer Sunday afternoon visit vividly. The first thing I noticed about Joann was that she was not dead. Five years out and cancer free, she looked healthy and wonderful—calm, reassuring, and full of information. "I am well and you can be too," is what she said to me and Don. A gift like no other—hope. Throughout all the evaluation and treatment Joann was available for support and to answer questions. I had lots of questions, like, "Is a one-centimenter lump really big or really little in the world of breast cancer?" Turns out it is more to the side of little than big.

Months later we decided to start this book.

Joann's Story

The mammograms I'd had for five years were fine, so I was horrified to discover a lump in my armpit. When something goes wrong, it's my style to run, not walk, to get things fixed, so I scheduled a mammogram right away. By the time I had the results and was told to have an ultrasound, it was a week later. We're sure it's nothing, they said. Don't worry, they said.

Ultrasound is interesting; the radiologist showed me a clear-ringed cyst and, behind that, a dense mass. The lump in my armpit was too high to see. Get a biopsy as soon as possible, he said.

To me that meant right then. I didn't go home; I drove straight to the gynecologist's office and said that I just knew he would want to see me. He did. Before I left there, I had an appointment with a surgeon to talk about a surgical biopsy. By that time another week would be gone. This time they didn't say don't worry.

I told myself I would *not* cry when I heard the diagnosis; I already know; let's just get going; but when the surgeon said I had cancer, a waterfall of despair washed over me, pouring from the roots of my hair down to the floor and covering my face with tears. Good for the surgeon, who put his hand on my shoulder to comfort me and said he'd be worried if I didn't cry.

My choices were not nice. They never are. (1) I could do nothing—for me, not a choice; or (2) I could attack this thing and have a mastectomy or a lumpectomy; whichever I chose, I would need both radiation and chemotherapy, because I probably had positive lymph nodes. I chose lumpectomy.

The surgeon said to make an appointment right away with a radiation oncologist and a medical oncologist. A what? We got some names. My husband called them from the surgeon's office.

Then I got on the phone. I lost my voice from talking. I wanted to be told people cared and that they thought I would be okay. I wanted help, help, any kind of help. I got it. All kinds of it. Best of all, my husband, Steve, was right by my side, every step of the way, supporting me, pushing me, crying with me. Without his help, it would have been so easy to give up.

✓ Checklist

❑   Start thinking about a personal care plan.

❑   Call your primary care physician or gynecologist.

❑   Find someone to go with you to the biopsy, as well as when you hear biopsy results.

❑   Determine who will organize your treatment/care—see an oncologist.

❑   Learn about your disease.

❑   Call helplines, such as American Cancer Society, National Cancer Institute, Susan G. Komen Breast Cancer Foundation, or Y-ME.

chapter 2

Riding the Emotional Roller Coaster

The words "cancer" and "malignancy" are very scary. When a
radiologist or your regular doctor suspects that you have cancer,
you get on what everyone describes as the emotional roller
coaster. It begins in the days before a biopsy or surgery, and its
ups and downs just go on and on. You may feel certain this is all
a mistake—"This can't be happening to me." A few minutes later
you may feel that your life is over. You might feel both at the
same time. Perhaps the most scary times are the times of
waiting: waiting for biopsy results, waiting for information about
lymph nodes, waiting to hear what your recommended treatment
will be. The reactions of shock, fear, anger, sadness, and dismay
are a necessary part in accepting that you are now a cancer
patient. That's tough to integrate with the many other aspects of
your identity, whether these be partner, mother, grandmother, or
grocery clerk, lawyer, or teacher, but accepting this piece of your
experience is essential. Acceptance of part of your identity as a
cancer patient will keep you alert to taking good care of yourself

and giving yourself the best possible opportunities to live to be a very old cancer survivor. It DOES NOT mean creating a new identity as a helpless person or an invalid. It simply means you have a diagnosis to integrate into your life, something like the way diabetics learn to make their life-threatening illness and treatment part of their lives. It can be done. No one can tell by looking at you that you have had cancer, and it is up to you who will know.

Another common reaction on hearing that you have cancer is "Why me?" The emotional ramifications of this depend on the answer you give yourself. Some answers may be as straightforward as knowing that breast cancer runs in your family and that you had a higher than normal risk. Or it can be more complicated. The answer to "Why me?"can be harmful to your feelings of self-worth. Answers such as "because I was a bad mother or person," or "because I haven't been good about getting mammograms," or "because I didn't breast-feed my child," or "because I haven't been going to church," or "because my sex life has been too active (or not active enough)," and probably lots of other ones, are characterized by feelings of guilt and fantasies of punishment. Psychologically, these beliefs can make sense because they tend to offer control. For example, if I believe that I got cancer because I wasn't being the kind of mother I thought I should be, then I can change and maybe this change will magically take away this punishment and save my life. The answers we give ourselves to "Why me?" are often the basis for the bargaining with God that sometimes happens: "Just let me get over this and I promise I will do . . . ."

The trouble is, we don't know why some women (and a few men) get breast cancer and others don't, and we *do* wonder "Why me?" We think, "If only . . .": If only I had had more frequent mammograms, or if only I had lost weight or exercised more, or breast-fed my children, or had a prophylactic mastectomy—and on and on. These thoughts are normal. They do, however, tend to focus on what is past and are critical and punitive rather than healing.

Remember that such thoughts are an effort to make sense of a confusing and painful experience. Try to redirect your energy to helpful, constructive thinking and planning. When you find yourself dwelling on negative thoughts, listen to some music, take a walk, make plans for your next stage of treatment, call a friend, or take any other positive, constructive action. If this doesn't seem to work for you, consider talking with a counselor or therapist who can help you let go of self-critical ruminations.

Having lots of different kinds of feelings and intense feelings is part of the territory, but they may lead to unhealthy behaviors. Not sleeping is one possible problem. Your mind may be unable to stop thinking about cancer, and you are worrying and worrying, even when it is time to go to sleep. Or maybe you can get to sleep, but you wake up at two, three, or four o'clock in the morning and can't get back to sleep because you are so terrified. If you have had to stop estrogen therapy abruptly upon suspicion of breast cancer, one of those drenching hot flashes may awaken you first, and then you start to worry. Sleep disturbance is likely to be temporary, but there is no reason you should continue to lie awake terrified in the middle of the night. If sleep disturbance becomes an issue, let your doctor know; the doctor can prescribe medications for short-term use to help with sleep and should assess whether you might be depressed.

People who are depressed are usually able to say they feel depressed, although not always. Does it feel like you are crying *all the time*? Sometimes a spouse, family member, or friend may recognize your depression first; if they express concern, listen to what they have to say and talk with your doctor. Sometimes depression is expressed as intolerable anxiety—nothing is ever going to be okay again, so what's next?—or as irritability—anger at everything and everybody all the time, with not an ounce of patience left. Have you completely lost your ability to concentrate on any story line more complicated than a cartoon? Maybe you don't care—about anything—you want to not feel so bad, and you just give up. Maybe you want to go to bed, pull the covers over your head, and never come out—and that is exactly what you have been doing. The future seems to have no meaning; getting through each day requires more energy than you have. And all of this is so unlike how you have always been. Any of these symptoms can be part of the pain and the ups and downs that result from a diagnosis of cancer or even side effects of some cancer treatments; however, when the symptoms are severe and come in combination with one another, there's a chance that you are suffering from a *treatable* depression.

In summary, the following symptoms should make you wonder if you are depressed:

- trouble sleeping or sleeping too much nearly every day;
- significant weight loss or gain accompanied by marked change in appetite;
- observable slowing in behavior (lethargy) or observable agitation (can't be still);
- fatigue or loss of energy nearly every day;
- feelings of worthlessness or extreme guilt nearly every day;
- inability to think, concentrate, or make decisions;
- recurrent wishes to die; and
- no interest in activities that you usually find pleasurable.

This list seems very tidy, and it misses any description of the depth of the despair and pain that so often is part of depression. All the feelings inside are so awful that it seems impossible to connect with the routine everyday concerns of others or to connect with your own life.

Depression is treatable; it can go away with talking therapy and antidepressant medication. To not treat depression just because it is predictable that someone with cancer might get depressed just does not make sense. To lessen your suffering should be one of your primary goals as well as that of your doctor. Don't accept a dismissal of your feelings by your doctor. Ask the doctor to go through your symptoms with you, make a list of them, and get some treatment for you. You can follow your symptoms and let your doctor know when they get better. Talk with your family about this as well; sometimes they'll know when your depression is getting better before you do.

These symptoms are probably more likely to occur in the beginning of the emotional process of dealing with a cancer diagnosis, but they can happen anywhere along the course of your treatment and even afterward. It is sometimes difficult to know if a sleep disturbance is primarily from hot flashes or from depression, or whether the fatigue is from radiation or chemotherapy or from recovering from surgery rather than depression, but depression carries with it such apathy, hopelessness, and despair, that if you feel that way, ask about getting an evaluation and some treatment. You do not have to be suffering from depression to benefit from talk therapy. You are sure to be frightened or anxious or down at times, and if you think talking with a therapist might help, give it a try.

The typical duration of depression for women with a recent breast cancer diagnosis is six to eighteen months. If you feel depressed, you may think there is something wrong if you are not "over it" in a month or two. It takes longer than this to recover from depression. Family members and friends also sometimes have trouble with this idea.

Other Aspects of the Emotional Roller Coaster and Emotional Integration

For months, or longer, every physical symptom—a cough, an ache or pain, or a little bump somewhere—brings back the BIG FEAR. This may be the same kind of fear you felt when you discovered your first symptom that did turn out to be cancer. Every symptom needs to be checked out with your doctor so that if it is a problem, you can get treatment, and if it is not a problem, then this can be one more step in the process of learning to trust your body again. For awhile, every trip to the doctor can feel like it will bring bad news.

Anxiety prior to every checkup is normal, even if this persists for years. Sleeplessness, restlessness, or trouble concentrating may make an encore throughout your treatment and recovery. Be extra kind to yourself. After your treatment is over, your friends will have relaxed and will be happy to see you pretty much back to your old self; they will have put your cancer behind you, but *you* will still be getting checkups every three months and getting scared every three months. Make sure a few especially important people in your life know how tough these times are so they can be there for you.

Ideas involving the future such as buying a new washing machine, buying a car, or taking a vacation may make you anxious. You may be thinking, "I can't plan that far ahead." That's normal too. Take your time. It may take a while before you can let yourself plan a trip until after you have had that next three-month checkup. Just start by planning one small trip at a time. Gradually you will once again be able to believe in and plan for the future. But don't lose your newfound ability to treasure and revel in every new day—the one you have right before you.

You may very well have to deal with normal developmental changes, such as menopause, at a not-so-normal time, because of the effects of chemotherapy. You may be too young to be going through menopause, and you will have plenty of feelings about this in addition to feelings about having cancer. You may already have gone through menopause and have been taking estrogen replacement, which you now have to give up, and it feels like you have to go through the whole thing all over again. Or, you may have been hoping you would finally get to menopause, and a positive side effect of having cancer treatment is getting rid of menstruation forever. The reactions are different for everyone.

There are all kinds of sexual and emotional adjustments to be made in yourself and in your relationships. Loss of hair with chemotherapy, fatigue with radiation therapy, loss or scarring of a breast with surgery, vaginal pain during intercourse caused by dryness brought about by menopause or treatment with tamoxifen—all of these can mess with your image of yourself and with your sexual functioning.

Other emotional adjustments involve your relationships with family members. We both dealt with feelings about our spouses if we were to die: Would he be able to cope? Would he remarry? We had questions about aging parents and children: Who would care for my mother if I die? What will happen to my kids? The answer to this is not to cross too many bridges. It is unlikely you are going to die in the next weeks or months, even though having cancer can make you think this way. Deal with these kinds of issues if they become a reality.

Yes, there is a lot to handle, but it can be done—unfortunately it is being done time and time again by thousands of American women each year. You can do it too. You can take care of yourself and address every single one of these problems.

Some Benefits Along the Way

You begin to understand that none of us lives forever—and that every single day and every single loving relationship is truly a gift. Your awareness and sensitivity to life's textures and colors and to its smell and feel can be heightened.

You may lose any fear you may have had about what to say to someone who has cancer or any other illness. You will make new friends. You will probably find that you are stronger and more resourceful than you ever thought before. You can be proud of how you are handling this challenge, and you are better prepared to accept others.

You should find new and wonderful ways of caring for yourself. Maybe you have never had a massage, or learned relaxation techniques, or learned to meditate. Maybe you never exercised regularly or never took the time for a bubble bath with a good book—every night—before this happened.

You will probably also learn how much you are loved through all the support and caring you receive from others—if you make sure to let them show it.

You have an opportunity to mend relationships that have been in bad repair—or you can come to an understanding that life is too short to stay in destructive relationships.

You may make some deeper discoveries, on your own or with the help of counseling or psychotherapy, about who you are and what you value, about ways that you can soothe yourself.

You may come to find new avenues for your creativity, and you pursue them—giving to others, writing, painting, poetry, cooking—there are lots of ways.

We believe all of these gifts are possible, but we don't think anyone should feel they have to be pleasant, courageous, attractive, and a "trooper" all the time. Often you will be a lethargic, gloomy grump, and that's okay too. Save your energy for what really matters.

What Can Help

1. Developing your own individualized care plan that you think about, construct, write down for yourself, and then follow faithfully. Elements that can be included are:

- Good nutrition: you feel better when your body gets what it needs;
- Rest: pay attention to how much you need, and adjust it appropriately;
- Exercise: schedule some every day;
- Water: drink plenty—at least a liter, preferably two, every day;
- Contemplative time/stress reduction—relaxation, meditation;
- Something you do for pleasure;
- Set your priorities every day, and learn to say no to unwanted demands;
- Set your priorities every day and learn to say yes to offers of help;

- Learn to ask for what you need;
- Let other people know how you wish to be treated—this includes your nurses, medical technicians, and doctors;
- Follow the medical regimen you and your doctor have decided is best for you; and
- Have patience with yourself and kindness toward yourself, especially when you can't do or be all that you want, or when things just don't go right.

2. The understanding of friends and family. You may have to invite this understanding by sharing your feelings and fears as well as listening to theirs.

3. Conversations with someone who has been there—another cancer survivor or in a support group of cancer survivors.

4. Counseling or psychotherapy, with or without medications, to optimize your emotional functioning.

5. Having fun when you can. The Diana Price Fish Foundation (303-639-9110) offers opportunities for fun for adults undergoing cancer treatment in the Denver area, including out-of-state patients who are in Colorado for their treatment. This is analogous to the Make-a-Wish Foundation for children, but is for adults. Unfortunately, so far there are no other such foundations nationally.

❏   ❏   ❏

Earlene's Story

Keeping a journal helped me through. This entry was from the 25th day after I learned my diagnosis:

"This writing is also about telling. I can't seem to stop telling. In some ways I think of it as being like a 12-step program. The first step for me is saying over and over 'I have breast cancer.' It has helped me grieve—crying and crying. I miss my life of the days before the diagnosis, I miss the way I used to experience myself, my body, and my identity.

"I have been so mad, I mean really ANGRY. I can see myself punching my fist through walls or smashing every dish in the kitchen.

"Last Sunday a couple of my close friends came to visit. I told them how painful the biopsies had been. Large needles had been pushed through both my breasts to snag pieces of tissue. I hated even the sight of the dress I wore that day. I couldn't imagine ever wearing it again. I wanted to rip it to shreds. So we did. My friends and I tore it to tatters. Then we threw all the pieces into a big metal bucket so we could burn it. My husband was watching this process, somewhat curious and somewhat bewildered. He got up from his desk and said, 'If you are going to burn it, let's do it safely.' He took the bucket to the back yard, soaked the shreds in charcoal lighter fluid, and then we torched it! All in all a very satisfying day."

Joann's Story

The emotional roller coaster took me for a stomach-dropping ride. Unfortunately, having cancer isn't like being in an amusement park. You can't get off the ride; you will probably have to ride again, even if you say you're not going to. And it's not fun.

Sleepless nights—like everyone, I had them. Usually they didn't become a problem, because most of the time I was so tired I would sleep anyway. The worst night was before I had a confirmed diagnosis. I hurt everywhere, my back, my mind, my heart, my soul. That night was endless. We were just trying to have a long weekend away. Even many miles away from Denver, we couldn't get away from the problem. The next morning, Steve called my doctor who prescribed a sleeping medication. Just knowing I wouldn't have to toss all night helped, and I hardly ever used it.

Depression—you can't help feeling low, but I didn't become clinically depressed. It's not clear why some people do and some don't, but I didn't have that to add to my troubles. I was just lucky.

Anger—yes, every time I went for chemotherapy. It surfaced for the first time so unexpectedly. At the end of the session with my oncologist during which she outlined my entire treatment protocol, she asked if I'd like to have my first treatment right then. I was so shocked and off guard that I could hardly respond, and even though there was a significant reason I wouldn't have that first treatment that day, by the time we got home I was ranting, raving. I flung my handbag across the garage floor, breaking stuff as I went.

Other family members ride the roller coaster, too, not just the patient. In our case, sometimes Steve and I were on opposite cars. Often when he was down, I was up, so we were able to help each other a bit better than if our reaction times had been the same. It's useful for significant others to be aware and take care of their own feelings. They may need help, too.

✓ Checklist

- ❏ Begin to develop an individualized care plan.
- ❏ Accept your identity as a cancer patient.
- ❏ Recognize the symptoms of depression.
- ❏ Look at possible benefits along the way.
- ❏ Invite the support of friends and family.
- ❏ Consider joining a support group.
- ❏ Have conversations with someone who has been there.
- ❏ Consider counseling or psychotherapy.

chapter 3

Friends and Family

During treatment for cancer you have to learn to ask for help when you need it. This chapter will be useful if you don't know what to say when a friend asks, "What can I do to help?" It's so easy to say you are okay and don't need anything, but most people who ask this really want to do something for you, and they would like it if you are able to tell them what will be most helpful. It is up to the patient, or to her significant other, to tell friends who've offered help in this way what is needed. Our list contains few surprises, but some of the ideas here will be communicated best by significant others. Let them know what of these things you might really like even if *you* don't want to ask for them.

Even though this may seem like an extra burden when you are already dealing with so much, you are the person who will have to help your friends and family know how to talk to you; you will have to decide how much you want to tell people about your disease; you will have to talk to your significant other about your needs, including sexual needs; and you will have to tell your children what is happening to you. If you do these jobs well, you will not have to worry about why no one is talking to you, or whether your children are frightened by not knowing what is

31

happening to you, or whether your significant other understands how to meet your sexual needs (or your lack of them).

Arranging for Company

You will need someone to go with you to appointments and treatments. Talk with your significant other or your friends ahead of time to arrange for this kind of help. Choose someone for these expeditions who would not have to bring along small children; at best children will be bored, confused, or tired and at worst frightened. Most important, you need someone who can concentrate on your needs. Choose a person you won't mind hearing intimate details or seeing your scarred body.

At the appointment, ask this person to go into the doctor's office or the treatment room with you. Although no one is allowed to be in the room with a patient receiving radiation treatment, if you are going for chemotherapy, you may find it comforting to have your friend sit by you during the treatment. This is not the assignment for anyone who is frightened by needles or procedures or who becomes dizzy or ill. Ask someone you are sure will follow through and be on time. Time pressures only increase your stress in an already stressful situation.

Visits and phone calls can also be comforting. Let your friends know when they can call or visit. Ask them to leave messages for you if you can't come to the phone, and say you will call them back when you are feeling stronger. They should be able to take their cues from you regarding the length of the call or visit. If you get tired, don't hesitate to tell them so and cut visits short.

Controlling Hospital Visits

Hospitalization happens when you have surgery, become especially ill, or need intensive treatment. If you are hospitalized, having visitors may be intrusive or just too tiring. Our rule of thumb is this: Ask friends not to come to the hospital unless you specifically request them to. They can send flowers, cards, or a magazine, but should wait until you are home before asking to visit. If they telephone when it is inconvenient or you are feeling unable to talk for any reason, just say so, and then hang up; tell them that just hearing from them lets you know they are concerned about you.

Letting Others Know Your Condition

Friends will want to know how you are. Choose one close friend as a contact person who will always know what's going on with you. How did your surgery go? What were the pathology results? Have your contact person call or talk to others about you rather than having everyone calling your significant other, who might have to repeat the information many times. You could even set up a calling pyramid if you have lots of friends to keep in touch with.

Talking to Friends: Talking to you about your illness may feel awkward for your friends, especially if they haven't had experience with death or serious illness. We encourage you to talk as openly as possible with friends and family, because if you can talk about the situation, usually they will find it easier to support you. Your behavior will let others know what to say. The first step is to let them know, just as matter-of-factly as if you'd said you have the flu, that you are being treated for breast cancer, with a comment or two about where you are in this treatment. Often they may ask a question, and if you respond as easily and honestly as you can, they will feel more comfortable and be willing to ask another time how you are.

Let people know it is all right to ask how you feel, but they should not expect a standard answer. Friends may be shocked or surprised by something you tell them about your condition, but we hope they can be supportive. If you share something about your treatment that has hurt or dehumanized you in some way, you should understand that this may be hard for them to hear, and they may not know how to respond. When you have felt especially hurt or dehumanized, the person to tell about this is your doctor. If it's been a bad day and you are feeling awful about something or would rather not talk, let others know in a way that is comfortable for you, but will not make them feel as if they are intruding. Thank them for asking about you, and tell them the truth. Don't say you're fine when you're not. You don't need to go into great detail if you don't want to, but refusing to acknowledge their interest isolates you from people who care.

Make a conscious decision about how you want to manage phone calls. Friends and relatives will be reassured that they are not intruding if you take responsibility for this. Don't answer the phone if you don't want to talk. Turn it off or unplug it when you are exercising, meditating, sleeping, talking with a guest—anytime you don't want to be interrupted.

Talking to Your Doctor: From the very beginning you need to feel that your doctors are on your team. Try to separate your feelings about the treatments they are recommending from who they are. Your need for treatment may make you angry (and likely will), but that is not your doctors' fault, and it will help you if you can be their partner in the treatment. Make a list of every question you have, take it with you, and get all the answers. There are no dumb questions. Your understanding of what's going on and your cooperation will make handling the treatment easier. Don't be worried about crying in front of your doctors. They'll understand.

Of course being treated for cancer is difficult, both physically and emotionally. Almost inevitably some little thing will happen to you during this time that can be so upsetting and angering, because you are already so upset by having cancer, that you don't know what to do with your feelings; if this anger goes on and on, it might be wise to consider talking with a therapist about it. However, if the anger arises because of a specific incident, you can help yourself and other cancer patients by bringing the problem to the doctor most closely involved. We both felt furious with (different) radiology technicians who ignored our feelings and pressured us thoughtlessly. We felt we couldn't let the circumstances go by and talked to the doctors, which helped us because we thought the problems would be solved.

When you are angry in this way, the best approach is not to yell and scream at "them" about what "they" did to you. Call the doctor's office as soon as you have your thoughts organized and ask to talk to the doctor. Even though doctors are often unavailable to talk to you when you call, they *will* call you back. Tell the doctor you've had a problem. Explain exactly what happened to you and how that made you feel. Your voice may shake, and you may cry again, but you need to do this so you have some sense of control over the situation. Focusing on your own feelings helps keep others from feeling attacked, and you will get your point across better. If you have a specific remedy in mind, say so, and ask the doctor to help you with this.

Talking to Children: This is one of the hardest things you will do, but you must do it, because children know instinctively when something is wrong with their caregivers. You do not need to involve them in frightening details or information that is over their heads, but honesty is so important. Judge what to say by their ages and by the questions they ask, but they are all sure to want to hear you say that you are not going to die. Unless your original diagnosis is dire, you are not likely to die at this point from either the cancer or its treatment. (If things change, you or someone will have to talk to them about that then.)

For all children, even small ones, you need to say that you have breast cancer. Giving the disease a name tells them it is not just an unknown bad thing, but rather that you and your doctors know what it is and how to treat it. If you are having surgery, say so. Tell them that you have a lump in your chest that the doctor will be cutting out so that it can't make you sick. You can show them as you talk approximately where that lump is (outside of your clothing, of course). If you are having radiation and/or chemotherapy treatment, you should tell them that the doctors will be giving you some medicines that may make you feel sick for a while, but that these medicines will be helping make you well. You can tell them you may lose your hair. Take your time. Do it in a setting that is comfortable and intimate so that they feel your love and care for them—don't tell them in the car on the way to a soccer game. Be sure to let them ask questions, and encourage them to come to you about whatever they want to know; if you don't, their imaginations can create scenarios much worse than anything that is really true.

Even when you talk openly with children, they can imagine that your illness is somehow their fault. For example, children can worry about awful consequences of times they've been angry with you. They probably won't ask, but be sure to let them know that the cancer is not their fault—it's *nobody's* fault.

You can be certain children will react to the knowledge of your illness; the nature of the reaction will depend on your children. Listen for cues from them and be prepared to have more than one talk. Do not be alarmed if young children in their reaction to their fear seem to lose recently acquired developmental achievements—for example, a $3\frac{1}{2}$ year old might start bed wetting. However, if a child has a particularly severe reaction—becomes extremely fearful, clingy, angry, difficult, sleepless, or quiet—consider asking for professional help.

What About Sex?

Sexuality and sexual intimacy are two different aspects of the effects of being treated for cancer. Both have significant effects on your life and should not be shoved under the rug.

Sexuality has to do with how you feel about yourself as an attractive and sexy person. In our culture, breasts are a prominent focus of sexuality, and the disfiguring changes that inevitably occur with treatment for breast cancer can be devastating to a woman's image of herself. Every breast cancer patient has to deal with these changes. Huge, ugly scars (or even small, not-so-ugly ones) may affect your arm movement, and you have to work hard in physical therapy to overcome this. You may elect to have reconstructive surgery in order to recover some of the femininity you feel you have lost. Most of us know about ordinary bad hair days and how they can affect self-image. The loss of hair during chemotherapy can make us feel like hiding. There are lots of assaults to our feelings about ourselves during this time. The deep-down worst feelings are these: Who would want to have sex with someone who looks like I do? Will anyone ever want to again? How can my partner want to touch me?

Your ability to deal with this may lie in the strength of your self-image prior to your diagnosis. If you have relied on your outward beauty to define you as a sexy person, you may need to work on believing that your real beauty is more than just the sum of your 2,000 pretty body parts. In the meantime, an attractive wig that looks like your own hair can do wonders. If you are daring, a new short-short hairstyle or even no-hair style will be uplifting. Maybe a collection of great hats and scarves will give you just enough pizzazz. Just knowing that you can have breast reconstruction may allow you to put off that worry for the time being. A makeover could give you a new, better-than-ever feel about how you look, one that carries over after your treatment is finished.

Most of the changes will last only a few months after treatment is finished, and then you will look like your same old self. Some of us may tattoo our scars with butterflies as a badge of honor that reminds us of how beautiful we are to have come through this treatment, while others may quickly have reconstructive surgery. If the way you look leads to real depression (see Chapter 2), then you should ask your doctors to help you deal with this.

Sexual intimacy during treatment can be a source of difficulty for couples. The most important factor in maintaining a stable sexual relationship any time is openness and good communication between partners about what each needs and what feels good, and this is especially true when one person is ill.

Some couples slide easily into a mutual understanding about each other's sexual needs and feelings, and if this is the case for you don't make it a problem. Several factors may contribute to some need for adjustments in having sex. After surgery, pain and stiffness cause discomfort, and your appearance may create embarrassment. During radiation and chemotherapy treatments, tiredness, illness, and general debilitation can cause you to lose interest in having sex. Hormone therapy using tamoxifen sometimes contributes to vaginal dryness and discomfort during intercourse, and if this occurs you should discuss this with your gynecologist or oncologist, because there are remedies such as local lubricants. However, these things may affect you not at all, and you may feel that having sex gives you a sense of well-being that helps you feel normal and loved. Whatever your individual case may be, you and your partner need to be talking about this.

Having one person in a relationship who is seriously compromised is difficult on the other person. That person may feel excluded, abandoned, ignored, or otherwise shoved aside unless the couple can come to understandings on when hugging is enough, or when intercourse can comfortably happen, or what each is able to do for the other, or when a normal relationship might resume.

An excellent resource is the American Cancer Society's *Sexuality & Cancer: For the Woman Who Has Cancer, and Her Partner.* Although it covers problems created by many different cancers, not just breast cancer, it has a lot to offer in terms of understanding what causes sexual difficulties and how to cope with them. This booklet is free: just call 1-800-ACS-2345. Another helpful (and free) resource for the partners of women being treated for breast cancer is Y-ME's pamphlet, *When the Woman You Love Has Breast Cancer.* Call 1-800-221-2141. This is also the number for the Y-ME Men's Hotline, a place where a man can ask to talk with a male volunteer. Unfortunately, we know of no analogous resource for lesbian partners; however, if you are in an area where gay and lesbian cancer support services are available, that would be the place to start.

Gifts

None of us likes to ask for gifts, but here are some suggestions that very close friends or significant others can suggest to acquaintances who would like to "do something" for you.

Food: We think cancer patients do better if they don't always have to eat their own cooking. For one thing, they probably don't feel much like preparing meals. For another, after using energy to fix food, they may not have the energy to eat it, or it may no longer seem appetizing. A casserole or a pot of soup or stew are on the time-honored list of comforting foods. Friends should understand that what they bring might not be needed immediately, so if the food can be frozen and saved for a particularly tough day, so much the better. Alternatively, groups of friends can plan (with your input) days when someone will bring in a meal—sometimes this can happen every week if you need it. If friends ask what to do for you, you can tell them to bring something for your family, if not for you. Mention that it would be helpful to have the food in disposable containers so you won't have to bother with returning them. Even if you don't think you need food, let people bring it anyway; you never know when you or your family will be too tired or preoccupied to make a meal. Getting food was one of the most helpful gifts we received.

Cards and Letters: This is one of the least intrusive ways anyone can let you know they are thinking of you. Earlene had one friend who sent a card every day during the last month of her radiation treatment—all funny ones. It is delightful to receive a kid's school picture, a cartoon, or a pressed flower. We each got lots of cards and letters, and every one brought a tear or a smile or both.

Prayers: If you want them, ask your minister, priest, rabbi, or other spiritual leader or teacher to have prayers said for you. Bible study and prayer groups would be pleased to add you to their prayers. If you are in such a group already, they may want to plan a special meeting for you. We heard of a group that encircled the home of a member with breast cancer, holding hands and praying for her—what a moving and uplifting thing to do.

Books, Tapes, and Videos: The best books are simple ones. We received all kinds, but we thought the best were photography books on the topics of smiles and kisses and books that made us remember to laugh. Books about cancer should be chosen carefully. They should contain messages of love and hope. Someone might consider giving you one of those lovely bound blank books to use as a journal.

Relaxation tapes in general can be helpful. A good friend gave Earlene a tape by Carl Simonton which she found invaluable. Not only did it bring a bit of peace, it also gave directions for meditating, emphasizing healing, and visualizing. Joann especially enjoyed receiving some tapes of Native American flute music.

If you have favorite, funny, or recent movies you might enjoy seeing, you could ask a friend to rent them for you (and return them); if you feel like having company, you could watch together. It's a good way to get your mind and conversation away from your situation and be with a friend at the same time.

Flowers: Flowers are always a lovely and thoughtful gift. Joann received a small bouquet every week for the six months of her treatment time. Flowers remind the patient that someone would like to brighten her day. This is one thing a significant other can suggest. You can even send flowers to yourself!

Extra Ideas—Mugs, T-Shirts, Chores, and Listening: One friend came up with a great idea—a big gift bag containing seven individually wrapped gifts, one to be opened at the completion of each of the seven weeks of radiation therapy. One of the gifts was an extra large, soft T-shirt with the words "I DON'T WANNA" written in large letters across the front. What a great shirt to wear to radiation or chemotherapy! Gifts that suggest a little rebellion are just fine.

If you have some favorite pastime such as working crossword puzzles or jigsaw puzzles, playing card games, reading detective or romance stories, drawing, painting (maybe no more complex than paint-by-number), crocheting or other crafts, a gift in that line might bring you pleasure. Playing card games or doing a craft with a friend can be a lovely diversion, but again, only if you feel up to it.

Your partner can tell friends that right now you won't write thank-you notes. While you will want them to know how much you appreciate what they've done, the number of notes you would want to write may be overwhelming. This isn't a time to stand on formality. Try to mention a gift from someone when you talk to them, but if you forget, they will surely ask if you received it.

As mentioned earlier in the book, there are special gifts for special times. We hope you can tell your friends about some of them. For Earlene, it was a close friend who washed and styled her hair the day she got home from the hospital after surgery. This friend was also good at polishing nails. For Joann, it was a small artificial Christmas tree from the school staff that arrived a month before Christmas, followed by an ornament each day in the mail, and trays of Christmas cookies from neighbors and friends who knew she wouldn't be baking anything that year. Another friend who "babysat" after a hospitalization brought a collapsible pyramid and crystals for her to lie under while listening to some favorite music.

Earlene's radiation therapist made her feel more like a fellow human being—and made her smile—every time he showed her a new photograph of his baby daughter. A gift certificate for a massage is wonderful. Sometimes the massage therapist is willing to come to the client's home—extra nice.

You might find the following ideas to be intrusive, so we want you to be able to respond honestly when you are asked about them:

- taking your kids for the day or an evening;
- washing a few loads of clothes and catching up on the ironing;

- asking you to go have a nap while they clean up the kitchen;
- asking you if you feel up to a very short walk;
- grocery shopping or doing other errands; or
- offering to do a massage.

The best gift of all is just having a friend who will listen to fears, worries, and successes. Friends don't need to feel they have to make everything all right—they can't. Whatever they can do is great.

For the Spouse or Significant Other: These people carry a huge burden. They do much of what the patient usually does, while doing their own jobs, keeping the family in balance, helping the patient get to treatments, and trying to maintain an optimistic, upbeat attitude. It can be awfully lonely to be doing everything, and people only think to ask about the patient. You can tell friends to support them, too. Friends can

- ask how they are feeling;
- offer to take over something they do;
- take them to lunch;
- let them know they are being thought about, too;
- watch for signs of depression in the significant others, and encourage them to get professional help if there seems to be a problem;
- ask them to do something they like to do that will take them away from responsibilities for a little while. Arrange for help for the patient during this time if it's needed; and
- bring food.

We've included a "wish list" page you can photocopy listing some of these ideas. You can cross out anything you don't want, add others you need (like someone to walk the dog when you can't), and pass the list on to family members and friends. They can coordinate the effort among themselves. After you read Chapter

4, you might want to add something from our suggested shopping list to your wish list.

What Friends Say

There is no doubt that well-meaning friends may say something that will cause you discomfort or anxiety. You need to understand that such things come from their concern for you and from a lack of understanding about how to help you. An example of this is their sharing stories about other people's treatments or outcomes, especially if the stories are not optimistic. It won't be helpful to hear about someone who may be having worse treatments than you; this won't make you feel any luckier about your own situation. You will need to let these things just slip away, remembering that you are different from everyone else—just because it happened to someone else does not mean it will happen to you.

A cancer patient feels isolated, abandoned by her body, and needs to feel that her friends and family will stand by her. It isn't unusual for those who can't cope to disappear, if not permanently, at least during the treatment phase. Welcome them back when they come; you'll be able to rely on others for the time being.

We hope your friends will make *brief* phone calls. They can say: "I've just been thinking about you and wanted to hear your voice." They can say: "I know you had a treatment today. I hope it went well." They can say: "Call me up when you want to talk." They can say: "I love you." That's all it takes.

❏   ❏   ❏

Earlene's Story

The week after the diagnosis was so difficult, and one of the most painful jobs was telling friends and family. In the days prior to temporarily closing my psychiatry practice, which was equally painful, I phoned my son, away at college, to let him know about the diagnosis and the surgery. I called my parents and my brother. They were all shocked and concerned. My brother went right to work and found all he could about my kind of breast cancer on the Internet. He was positive and reassuring both to me and to my parents. I asked my son to come home after the surgery and he came, offering as always his wonderful smile and great sense of humor. He wanted to know exactly how radiation treatments worked, and he drove me to a couple of the treatments before he had to go back to school. Friends, family, colleagues—everyone—pitched in. I've never been so scared or received so much love and support.

Joann's Story

In talking to my third graders about my disease and treatment, I was as simple and honest as I could be with them. It turned out that the day I decided to talk to them was my last day of teaching, so I was glad I hadn't put it off any longer. They were prepared for my possible absences, but I hadn't anticipated that my first one would be long term. They wrote me letters about their feelings, and I did come to visit them a few times so they could see firsthand that I was really still a part of their lives. I was wearing a wig much of that time, but after I returned to work I decided I couldn't stand the wig any longer—I cut off what little hair I had and told them this was my Sinead O'Connor look, the no-hair look she wore then. Although they seemed shocked at first, they soon told me they liked my new cut, but they were insulted because I hadn't told them I had been wearing a wig.

Things Friends Can Do to Help

Go along to treatments or doctors' appointments

Bring food
- ❏ Treats for my family
- ❏ Meals to freeze for a bad day

Call me on the phone
- ❏ Ask how I'm doing today
- ❏ Listen
- ❏ Tell me you care
- ❏ Do a calling list if I'm hospitalized
- ❏ Understand if I'm unable to talk

Send cards or letters

Suggest or bring books helpful to recovery or having humor

Help with chores
- ❏ Grocery shopping
- ❏ Light housekeeping
- ❏ Babysit my kids
- ❏ Visit my aging parent

Visit at home if I'm well enough
- ❏ Share common interests
- ❏ Watch a movie with me
- ❏ Go for a walk with me
- ❏ Bring lunch or dinner and eat it with me

Help partners
- ❏ Invite them to lunch
- ❏ Ask how *they're* doing
- ❏ Go with them for an activity such as golf, tennis, shopping, a movie—just for a break
- ❏ Offer to do something they've taken on for me
- ❏ Offer to stay with me while they do something they want or need to do

Other: _____

_____

✓ Checklist

- ❏ Think of some ways friends can help you—give them the list.
- ❏ Let people know they can talk to you.
- ❏ Say "yes" when you can.
- ❏ Say "no" when you need to.
- ❏ Talk to your doctor when you feel hurt or dehumanized.
- ❏ Designate an information person.
- ❏ Talk to your children.
- ❏ Communicate openly with your spouse about both of your needs.

chapter 4

Shopping List

"When the going gets tough, the tough go shopping."

This time you have an excuse. There are some things you need. A friend once said, "When you're diagnosed with cancer, the first thing you do is buy all new underwear."

Actually, however, the first thing you really need is a **small cassette tape recorder with earphones,** because people, especially your doctors, will be saying lots of things you will need to remember. Even if you bring your spouse or a dear friend to your appointments, neither of you will remember everything—maybe only a small fraction of what is said. There is just too much to take in, much of what they say will be unfamiliar to you, and you are in shock. Record what your doctors say; also, you might want to record questions as you think of them to ask at your next appointment. Later on, you might want to use it for meditation or for soothing music during treatments. Don't forget the **blank tapes.**

Soft, moldable **cold packs** that can be chilled in your freezer cost less than $5 at most discount stores. Cold packs feel good and help reduce swelling after surgery. You can put ice cubes in plastic bags, but the edges of the cubes may be uncomfortable, and neither of us were able to devise a way to keep the bags from leaking. A cold pack is the answer to ice water in the sheets.

Here's where the new underwear really does come in. You may not want a bra at all after surgery, but if you have had a lumpectomy you might still want some support. The skin around the surgery and under the arm will be sensitive, so underwires or tight elastic are not good ideas. **Soft cotton bras** will also be useful if you will be having radiation therapy—they are just more comfortable. Mastectomy patients should discuss with their doctor what they should do about wearing a bra, particularly if you are heavy-breasted and uncomfortable not wearing one to support your remaining breast; a Reach to Recovery volunteer or a hospital employee trained to do this should visit you in the hospital to show you bras and **prostheses** (artificial replacements). If you opt not to wear a bra, **cotton undershirts** may make you feel more covered.

Cotton pads or **large cotton balls** will feel good over the surgery scar or under the tubing of the drain when you do want to wear a bra—not so much rubbing. If you are having radiation treatment, your therapist will tell you what you can't use—such as deodorants containing aluminum zirconium tetrachlorohydrex (an ingredient in most antiperspirants) or talc and perfumed skin creams—and what you can use, such as **aloe vera gel** and a deodorant powder made from **cornstarch and baking soda.** Soothing and moisturizing aloe vera helps heal irradiated and burned skin; you may be able to find it in a pump bottle. Look in health food stores for crystal salt rocks to use as a deodorant (not an antiperspirant), or see if you can order from a pharmacist a new nonmetallic deodorant called Altra. If you can't find either of these, make your own deodorant powder of equal parts cornstarch and baking soda. You can make it pretty by putting it in a nice dish or bowl with a fluffy powder puff on top.

Buy an **electric razor,** because after removal of lymph nodes you don't want to risk nicking any skin under your arms. Underarm numbness caused by surgery increases this risk. Using an electric razor reduces the risk of cuts you might get elsewhere that could bleed profusely if you are having chemotherapy.

A **lip moisturizer** is a must if you don't routinely use it. Hospitals are really dry places, and this will help when you are there. Plain Vaseline is also soothing for your lips if you develop any mouth sores during chemotherapy.

Some sort of soft **warm-up suit** that you can wear to radiation treatments or to doctors' appointments is awfully nice, because these are comfortable and you can get in and out of them easily. For radiation, it is helpful to wear something that buttons or zips up the front; pullovers can be a problem if you have difficulty lifting your arm. For chemotherapy treatments, you may also want to wear front-buttoning blouses, especially if you have a **port** (a special I.V. that usually remains in place between treatments); otherwise, something comfortable and loose-fitting will feel the best and will also look super if you don't want to wear a bra.

When you shop, read the labels of any health food supplements, any vitamins, any creams or deodorants, or anything you consider putting on or in your body. The simplest things are the best. Ask your doctor if you need any special treatments for your hair, or whether you need to be taking any extra vitamins, or if there are any special kinds of foods that will be helpful. If you can't sleep, talk to your doctor instead of taking whatever your friend might recommend. Your friends all want the best for you, but it may not be best to use anything that might contain any hormones. (If your tumor is not receptor-positive, and you will read about this later, this doesn't apply.) Just thank them for their help, talk with your doctor, and decide for yourself.

If you're planning to have chemotherapy, one possible side effect is hair loss. It's a good idea to visit a wig shop that specializes in helping cancer patients—your doctor can suggest one. Pick out a wig that is close to your natural color and style and arrange for the shop to hold it if you decide you want it later. Do it now so that if you do lose your hair, you have already chosen the color you want. Also, ask about special caps to help the wig stay in place; otherwise, you will be trying to depend on your last remaining strands of hair to pin it to, and this doesn't work very well. If your financial situation won't let you buy a wig, check out Y-ME's wig bank, or borrow one from the local chapter of the American Cancer Society. Also, look at the American

Cancer Society's TLC catalog for headcovers—scarves, hats, turbans in case you don't want to use a wig.

An antibiotic cream will help protect your skin from minor infections. This is particularly important for the arm and hand on the side where your surgery has occurred. Use it as your cuticle cream of choice, now and ever after, since infections can be a source of lymphedema (a buildup of fluid in your arm that can happen any time after the removal of axillary lymph nodes).

Waiting-room distractions are something you'll want to consider having with you. You will spend a lot of time waiting. By the time you finish your treatment, you'll have seen every magazine dating from 1990 on in every waiting room. Perhaps you are too agitated or tired to read anyway—take along some kind of handwork or your meditation tapes.

Remember, all of this is to make you feel more comfortable. None of these things should take much energy, time, or money to buy. If you have a choice between practical and pretty, choose pretty. Choose soft, choose warm. Make yourself feel good.

❑   ❑   ❑

✓ Checklist

❑   Cassette recorder and tapes
❑   Cold packs
❑   Cotton balls or cotton pads
❑   Soft cotton bras and/or T-shirts
❑   Aloe vera gel
❑   Cornstarch and baking powder deodorant
❑   Lip moisturizer
❑   Warm-up suit
❑   Read labels of all products you use.
❑   Pick out a wig if you think you might want one later.

chapter 5

Meditation and Relaxation

Several times we have recommended meditating as a way of helping yourself during this stressful time in your life. "Well," you say, "I don't know how to do that—I don't know anyone who's ever done it. How can I learn?" You might have a picture in your mind of saffron-robed monks droning *om* to the sound of temple bells. Really, meditation isn't that at all. Meditation is finding a quiet time and place to let go of the cares of daily life. It is centering and restful. It is simply a tool you can use to balance your inner self.

Deep relaxation is similar to meditation, but it is more a physical process; its goal is to leave the body feeling relaxed by creating tensions that you then let go. You will no doubt feel tense, and you can use deep relaxation alone or in conjunction with meditation.

What You Need

This is another time you need a cassette player with headphones. At first it is helpful to use a meditation tape that guides your thoughts in a positive way toward healing your body and teaches you how to concentrate and visualize. There are

53

many such tapes. (You can use CDs in place of tapes if you prefer—they may actually be more readily available.) We particularly like "Mindfulness: Meditation in Everyday Life," by Jon Kabat-Zinn; "Cancer Recovery and Recurrence Prevention," by Carl Simonton; and "Eight Meditations for Health," by Andrew Weil, M.D. As you become more adept at meditating, you might prefer to use tapes of simply the sounds of nature—birds, the wind, the ocean—or your favorite quiet music.

Meditating—What You Do

1. Pick a time (or preferably times) during the day when you plan to meditate for 20 or 30 minutes. Turn on your telephone answering machine, or just unplug the phone. Let your friends know you won't be available during these times. Early morning is a good time for one session, before the rest of the world is moving, or just after your children are off to school. A second time may be harder to find; you just have to allot it and stick to it.

2. Pick a comfortable place where you won't be interrupted. Sit where you can't hear messages if your phone rings. Be where you can look out at a favorite view or in a peaceful place for you or where the sun can shine on you. Joann's favorite spot was a window seat where the early morning sun washed over her. Earlene loved being outside on her deck.

3. Put on your headset and set the tape, ready to go.

4. Sit in a comfortable position—you need to find what works best for you. There are two traditional meditative poses: sitting upright on the floor on a cushion or folded blanket with your legs crossed, your hands resting gently on your knees, palms turned up to receive energy; or lying on your back on the floor, legs slightly apart, arms slightly away from your body, palms facing up. (You can bend your knees and let them fall gently together if lying on your back is hard for you.) You might want a light blanket to cover yourself if you choose the prone position.

Positions for Meditation

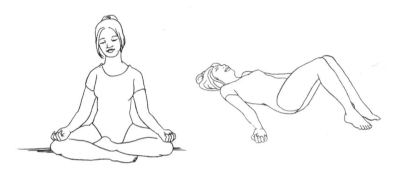

Figure 5.1   *The sitting and prone positions for meditation.*

5. Turn on the tape. If you are listening to a spoken tape, let your mind quiet itself by concentrating on the voice and the words. Then focus on your breath, simply noticing how it moves in and out of your body. If your mind wanders to other thoughts, bring it back to this quiet state by concentrating again on your breath and the voice on the tape. At first you may feel a little silly, but as you get used to the taped voices and the visualization exercises, daily meditation becomes something you will use more than at set times during the day. The techniques you use to let go of random, everyday thoughts during meditation can be used during whatever treatments you are having or at 2 A.M. when you wake up and your mind's wheels begin to turn.

6. Close your eyes. Later you can meditate with your eyes open if you choose, but at first if you look down and let your eyelids drop, it is easier to shut out unwanted and distracting images and to concentrate on your breath and the light behind your eyelids.

7. By concentrating on your breath, keep gently letting go of unhealthy thoughts (you know those, they're the ones that make you anxious and despairing and tearful). Simply note any stray thoughts and refocus on your breath. As you do this, it becomes easier to let in the healing thoughts. We both found the yellow warmth of sunlight helped bring us peace and healing.

8. When you leave a meditative state, do it slowly and deliberately, taking care to open your eyes only when you are ready and to move gently at first. Then, as you begin your normal activities, try to remember and reclaim the feeling of calm you have experienced in meditation. You can get it back at any time.

Especially if you have chosen the prone position, you may drift into sleep. Although sleep is not meditation, if you sleep you must need to, so don't criticize yourself if this happens. It's important to remember that this is a skill you will learn through practice, and it's okay if sometimes you can't let go of unwanted thoughts or problems; just realize that each time you sit to meditate will be different and will be what you need right then.

Deep Relaxation—What You Do

You can use deep relaxation to relieve tensions; this can be done a number of ways, but an easy way to do deep relaxation is as follows:

1. Get out that tape recorder or CD player, and put in some peaceful music of your choice.

2. Lie on your back on the floor, with your legs slightly apart, arms slightly away from your body. If this position isn't comfortable for you, put a pillow under your knees to relieve any stress on your lower back. You might prefer to lie on a mat or on carpet rather than on a hard floor.

3. Close your eyes. Touch your tongue lightly to the roof of your mouth, and let your jaw relax slightly, but keep your lips closed.

4. Do an inventory of your body; you can start with your feet and work up toward your head. Tighten the muscles of your feet and legs, and hold this position as tightly as you can for a few seconds. Then just let all the tightness go in that part of your body. Concentrate on creating this tightness and letting go for every muscle in your body. When you finish with your face and head, you are ready to give in to deep relaxation.

5. Breathe deeply for a few minutes, then let your breathing return to normal. Just lie there, letting the music wash over you for another 15 or 20 minutes.

6. As with the meditative state, gradually and gently bring your thoughts and your body back to normal. Wiggle your fingers and toes, rock your head slowly from side to side, and return the energy to the rest of your body.

If you need them, a light blanket over you may keep you warm, and a cloth over your eyes will shut out any light. After you learn to do this, you may find you prefer silence to the music. Use what works for you.

We have both found that throughout our healing, whether we are at five months or five years, meditation helps us when hairy thoughts come in the night or when our minds turn ordinary aches and pains into terrible things; deep relaxation helps when our bodies need respite.

❑　　　❑　　　❑

Earlene's Story

When I was 19, I learned transcendental meditation as one of the rites of a 1960s college student. The initiation ceremony was lovely—quiet room, candles, and a teacher who imparted to me my mantra, my secret meditation word. Despite my awareness of how valuable meditation is, I practiced it only sporadically. When I was diagnosed with breast cancer, meditation became an essential ingredient in my daily care plan. A good friend gave me Carl Simonton's "Cancer Recovery and Recurrence Prevention" tape. I listened to it twice a day for months. I don't believe that meditation or visualization can stop or cure cancer, but I don't think it hurts to be reminded of the healing power of our bodies. Getting cancer is a big glitch, but most of the time our bodies take care of weird cells, infections, and trauma. This tape helped me be grateful that my body had contained the cancer as well as it had—that my body would recover from the surgery and the radiation. Listening to the tape aided in a much-needed attitude adjustment and helped enormously with my anxiety. Most of the time I no longer need to hear a voice to help me, and I practice meditation silently at least once a day, usually after my morning walk. When I open my eyes after meditating, the world seems brighter and shinier.

Joann's Story

In 1978 I discovered yoga and had been practicing for many years before my diagnosis. When a friend brought me an audiotape called "Tropical Ocean," a subliminal healing tape from the Institute of Human Development in Ojai, California, I began to use it for daily meditation. Throughout my treatment I used many kinds of tapes, from sounds of nature to American Indian flute music to a choral setting of Psalm 121, as part of my own treatment plan. Sometimes absolute silence worked well for me. The yellow warmth of the morning summer sun felt especially curative, and I would sit there in meditation for a long time each day.

Always I took some of these tapes to listen to during my hour-long chemotherapy treatments. Even though Steve sat by my side through each one, he never minded that I seemed to peacefully "disappear" during this time. I hated the treatments and meditating during them helped me tolerate the process better.

✔ Checklist

☐   Choose meditation and relaxation tapes.
☐   Select a good time and place to meditate daily.
☐   Stick to your schedule—don't accept phone calls.

chapter 6

Surgery

Surgery is usually a key part of the treatment of breast cancer. Although the type of surgery and the care following surgery vary from individual to individual, the most common surgical interventions are lumpectomy or mastectomy. Your surgeon should be able to help you think through the decision about which is best for you. With either of these procedures, an axillary lymph node dissection is usually performed at the same time to detect any possible spread of the cancer.

Lumpectomy

Lumpectomy is the removal of the cancerous lump and enough surrounding tissue to obtain clean margins; that is, the area around the lump does not contain any cancerous cells. This surgery conserves as much of the breast as possible and is virtually always followed by radiation therapy to destroy any distant cancerous cells that may have escaped from the tumor. Additionally, breast surgery for cancer may be preceded or followed by chemotherapy, depending on the judgment of your physicians about the possible spread or kind of cancer you have. The surgeon may be able to remove as much as one-fourth of the breast (quadrantectomy) and still preserve your breast; if the area to be removed will be highly disfiguring anyway or for other considerations such as the size or type of your tumor or multiple tumors, the surgeon may recommend a mastectomy.

Mastectomy

Fortunately for us all it has become a priority for surgery to be as uninvasive as possible. Even forty years ago the standard surgery for breast cancer was a radical mastectomy, in which the breast tissue, chest muscles, and lymph nodes were all removed, as well as much of the skin, which was sometimes replaced by a skin graft. Today most mastectomies performed are the kind called modified radical mastectomy, in which breast tissue and lymph nodes are removed, but as much of the chest muscle and nerves as possible are retained. Although this is much less difficult surgery for the patient than radical mastectomy, sometimes there is nerve damage resulting in loss of feeling. Simple mastectomy, which is removal of breast tissue only, does not involve removal of lymph nodes. This kind of mastectomy may be used prophylactically to prevent cancer in a currently uninvolved breast.

Breast Reconstruction

If you have decided to have a mastectomy, you may wish to consider having breast reconstructive surgery. Women decide to do this for many reasons: They want their clothes to hang well and do not want to be bothered with a temporary replacement worn inside a bra; they want to look as much like they did before surgery as possible; they are young and/or not in a stable personal relationship and feel having no breast is a detriment to forming such relationships; and there are many other reasons.

At the time you choose a mastectomy, it is important to speak with a plastic surgeon right away if you think you may want a breast reconstruction either now or at some future time. This surgeon specializes in correcting deformed body parts and will work closely with your breast surgeon in determining how much tissue will be left behind to use for the reconstruction. If you decide to have breast reconstruction as part of your mastectomy surgery, you will be in the care of this team of doctors: The breast surgeon performs the mastectomy, and the plastic surgeon then takes over to do the reconstructive part. As you can imagine, this two-part surgery is lengthy and involved—be sure to ask how long this will take. However, the flip side is that you will not need a second surgery and subsequent recovery similar to what you will have with the mastectomy. However, later surgeries will be needed to put in a permanent implant and for the nipple construction.

You will be offered several kinds of reconstructive options, which fall into two basic categories—implants and flap reconstruction. Implants can be either a silicone envelope filled with saline or a silicone gel–filled implant. Both implants are likely to need replacement at some future time. There has been a lot of controversy, not to mention lawsuits, surrounding the safety of silicone breast implants. Today many plastic surgeons feel there is no safety problem with these implants and in fact may prefer them to the saline-filled type. This will be an issue for you to look into and consider as you think about reconstruction. The saline implants seem to need replacement sooner than the silicone implants. Whichever kind of implant you choose, an expander will be inserted under the chest muscle to make space for the implant, so have your plastic surgeon explain fully and in great detail how this is done. You need as much information as you can get in order to make the best choice for you.

Flap reconstructive surgery uses your own body's tissues to create a new "breast." TRAM flap surgery uses the transverse rectus abdominus myocutaneous tissues, which means abdominal muscle and fat tissues—a "tummy tuck." Other areas of the body may be chosen instead, such as muscle from the back, especially if you are thin and do not have enough abdominal fat. Each of these surgeries takes longer than implant surgery and involves more incisions than just the one on your breast. They also require a longer recovery time. You need to see pictures of the scars created by this kind of surgery and ask about abdominal and other muscle limitations that may be caused by flap reconstruction. The positive aspect of this kind of surgery is that nothing "foreign" is being put into your body.

If you are thinking about reconstructive surgery using implants, take a look at *Dr. Susan Love's Breast Book,* pages 387–401, for an excellent description of some of the options. Also, contact the Food and Drug Administration's Breast Implant Information Service at 1-888-463-6332. This is a lot of extra information to process when you are dealing with getting rid of your cancer, but it will be worth knowing in order to make informed choices.

Hospital Considerations

If you are like we were before we went to the hospital, your head is in a spin. We would like to help you not have to think of *everything* for yourself. We are assuming you will have at least an overnight stay in the hospital. However, some physicians regard lumpectomy and mastectomy as potential outpatient procedures. Be sure you have good home support and contingency plans in case of problems if you opt for an outpatient procedure.

1. What to Wear to and from the Hospital: The idea is comfort and ease of getting in and out of your clothes. A warm-up suit would work great. If you don't have one, remember these: comfortable soft blouse or shirt; slip-on slacks or skirt; and slip-on shoes (no bending over and tying).

2. What to Take to the Hospital:

A close friend or loved one: This must be someone you don't mind seeing you throw up or poorly covered in a hospital gown. They must know how to hold your hand or hug you if you need it. Tell this person your visitor policy. They must be willing to leave if you ask them to.

Your own pillow: Hospital pillows feel like bricks. Besides, your pillow smells like home.

Favorite blanket or afghan: This is familiar and adds warmth to what may look and feel like a pretty cold room.

A twin-size egg crate mattress: The hospital mattress may also feel like a brick. Especially if you are thin, your bones will like the extra comfort, and the nurses should be glad to put it under your sheet. If you don't have one, the hospital will be able to provide one. Ask for it right away.

A cassette recorder and tapes: You may not have the energy to read, so a relaxation tape, music, or a story may be soothing to you. If you feel like reading, have someone bring you a book or magazine, or even a crossword puzzle from the newspaper.

A change of underwear and socks: In case of an automobile accident on the way home—bad joke—sometimes black humor will seem like the only sense of humor available.

Toothbrush/toothpaste/small mouthwash: Tastes and feels better than what the hospital has. Be careful about the mouthwash if you're having chemotherapy—you may want to pass on that.

Whatever makes you feel good: (Here are some suggestions)

- Your own towel
- Brush and comb
- Lip moisturizer for your lips: Hospitals are really dry places.
- Glasses or contact lenses with case and solution
- *Cosmetics:* If a little lipstick or other makeup helps you feel better, take it.
- *Comfort items:* A teddy bear, a picture of someone who loves you, your good luck charm, or a religious token
- *A lightweight robe (optional):* Hospital gowns don't always close well in the back, and you may feel more comfortable getting out of bed if you have one to throw over your shoulders.

Don't forget your insurance or Medicare card.

3. What You Don't Need to Take:

Jewelry: Leave everything at home, including your wedding rings.

Money: You don't really even need a purse.

Nightgown or pajamas: You may want pajama bottoms, but you will have an I.V. line in one arm and the drain will be under your other arm, so it is almost impossible to change from the hospital gown after surgery.

4. Have These Things When You Get Home from the Hospital:

- SOFT cotton bra or undershirt
- Cold pack
- Cotton pads or large cotton balls

Your Condition

Remember that in the chapter on dealing with friends and family we suggested designating a caller to keep your many friends informed about how your surgery went. Be sure you've done that.

Feelings

Everyone is scared before going to surgery. We all react to being scared in different ways. The spectrum of reactions to fear include crying, shaking, wanting to run away, wanting to crawl under the bed and never come out, whining, becoming mad and irritable, longing for old comforts (things or people), becoming logical, intellectual and unaware of fear. Sometimes the fear is not felt until the scary event is over. Some know there is fear but try consciously to put it aside and focus on essential practical matters. Some never want anyone to see them cry. None of these ways is right or wrong; what often happens is that we have all of these reactions at different times and in different situations. How have you been feeling and expressing your fear? Make a list in your mind. You will probably notice how those around you are expressing their fear. We hope you can talk about yours.

Make a list of what scares you. Some of the things that come to mind may seem childish or silly. Remember, emotionally, we all become childlike in the face of illness and frightening procedures. We have included the following list of fears because sometimes it is tough to know what you are afraid of; naming the fear is the first step to addressing it. These are some of the most common fears:

Going under general anesthesia: If you are afraid of having a mask over your face, tell your anesthesiologist. It is fairly standard procedure to give you some medicine intravenously to help you relax and fall asleep before you ever get to the operating room.

Losing control—they will do something you haven't agreed to: The words you use with the surgeon should go something like this: "Please describe what you will be doing. What are the risks? Is there any way that you will be doing any kind of surgery while I am asleep that we have not discussed?"

What they will find—afraid the cancer is widespread: Believe me, we know this fear. Try to remember what has helped you feel less afraid in very scary situations in the past. Is that way of calming or comforting yourself appropriate now? Listen to your cancer recovery tape for calm and reassurance. Remember that there are many treatments available no matter what is found and that you will get those treatments.

How you will look after the surgery: This will vary according to the type of surgery you have. Lumpectomies can leave only a small scar, especially if the tumor is located where it and the lymph nodes can be removed through a single incision. If you are going to have a single or double mastectomy, ask the surgeon to describe how your chest will look after surgery. Ask about reconstruction options: You should know about these possibilities even if you elect not to have any reconstruction, and the plastic surgeon should show you pictures of reconstructions, even though these may not look exactly like you. Regardless of the kind of surgery you have, it is a loss. We grieved and we cried for the loss of our unscarred chest and for the loss of our health. You deserve to be sad and to grieve.

Being alone: Let someone know. Do everything you can to find someone you trust to go to the hospital with you and stay with you when you get home. It may be that you need to go stay with someone after you leave the hospital, if there is no one at home for you.

Being in pain: There is no reason to be in pain. Tell your surgeon that this is a fear. If you have pain when you are in the hospital, tell your nurse. Today many hospitals attach a delivery system for pain medication to your I.V., allowing you to manage pain relief yourself. Just knowing you can take care of this when you need to is reassuring. Some pain medications may make you sick at your stomach. If this happens, the doctor can give you a different kind of pain medicine or something to alleviate the nausea. There are solutions to this problem, but you may have to be persistent in asking for them.

Being a bad patient: Maybe you are afraid that you ask too many questions, or are embarrassed that you can't remember what the doctor or nurse said, or think you are silly or stupid for having your feelings, or feel you might be expecting too much attention from the nurses or doctors. Don't be. There is no such thing as a bad patient—there are plenty of scared patients, but no bad ones.

Death: We are all afraid of dying. You are not alone. Start thinking now of talking with someone—perhaps a rabbi, a minister, a friend, a therapist, a spouse or partner, or other family member. A support group may help. A few things are clear: A diagnosis of cancer is not a death sentence, and you are not dead now. You are doing everything you can to help your body. It is *extremely unlikely* you will die from surgery.

The fears listed above are examples of short-range fears. Try to stick to dealing with them, because they offer plenty of challenge by themselves. You should do anything you can to make your list shorter. The best way to shorten the list is to have a plan to address your fears in a helpful way. If you can, talk to someone about your fear; even if it doesn't go away at least you are not alone with it. Also, keep this rule in mind: You must treat your fears with kindness and sympathy. You must approach your own fears with the same concern you would those of your best friend or your own child—gently. It is *highly likely* your surgery will go just fine.

Your list will probably include other fears. Some are what we call long-range fears. One such fear results in being preoccupied with how you would deal with losing your hair if you have to have chemotherapy and if you lose your hair. There are usually a lot of "ifs" in long-range fears. You may never have to have chemotherapy and you may never lose your hair. We think about these things so much because they are concrete problems we feel we might have some chance of solving in the face of losing control over so much.

Physical Therapy

Do not go home from the hospital until you have met with a physical therapist and he or she has shown you how to do some exercises to stretch and strengthen the underarm area damaged by surgery. These are essential to good healing and regaining full range of motion in your arm. One immediate benefit from doing the exercises, which mainly involve stretching, will be if you plan to have radiation therapy following surgery. Having a good range of motion will help you get your arm in the correct position comfortably for the simulation and treatments.

❑   ❑   ❑

Because we had no personal experience with mastectomy and reconstruction, we asked a friend if she would share her story. Here it is:

Ruth's Story

At first, no choices were presented to me. It was, you have to have a mastectomy, so I went through the whole system, including seeing a plastic surgeon. My husband and I spent hours in the hospital getting all set up for mastectomy, but then I got another opinion. The second doctor said there was another choice—I could do the chemotherapy first. That's what I did. After that I had a lumpectomy. The next thing was supposed to be radiation, but the surgeon said that she felt the better, safer, and more conservative thing to do in my case was to have a mastectomy instead of radiation. And I said, "When can I go down and have it? I want to go down there tomorrow." I think for me it was easier because I'd already gone through this whole mastectomy scenario, so it wasn't a huge shock.

All the doctors said to me—because of my particular diagnosis—they would not object if I wanted to have the other breast removed at the same time. The real reason to do that is psychological, but it's like everything else, you have to sort it out for yourself. I asked for and had an MRI because I said I didn't want to hear that I would need a second mastectomy in six months—I really didn't want to hear that. I wanted to do it right then. The MRI was fine, and I ended up just doing the one side.

There were three weeks between the two operations [the lumpectomy and the mastectomy with reconstruction]. I had constant pain with the lumpectomy, much more than with the mastectomy. One thing that helped me tremendously was taking *Arnica montana* when I was having soreness. I needed painkillers both those two times, but they had to cut me off the painkillers because I *loved* painkillers so much. I would not come downstairs if the painkillers were upstairs.

We'd talked about reconstruction, and the doctors presented everything—it was actually hilarious. They said I could have a saline implant or a silicone implant or this

70

TRAM flap. TRAM flap, I thought, that's what I want, so I ended up in a little examining room with about five doctors grabbing my stomach, and I didn't have enough fat on my stomach. Everybody wanted to check with everybody else to see if I did—and I didn't. At that point they asked what *did* I want? They told me I could go to California where they can take it out of your butt, your shoulder, whatever they do, and they also talked about a long recovery time. For the TRAM flap they'd take muscle from my stomach and maybe I wouldn't be able to sit up correctly—I thought, I don't want this, so I'll try this saline thing. I didn't want the silicone implant even though my plastic surgeon was very prejudiced toward it; supposedly it looks a lot better and it feels better to the touch. The saline shows ripples in your flesh, because it's water in a bag, but three or four ripples don't bother me. I kept telling them, "Look, I'm into good enough." They couldn't believe it. You know, when you decide on reconstruction, part of you is going "Why am I doing this? I know it's not going to look like my other one, but I want to look good in clothes, have symmetry, and so I can have something that's good enough if my daughter sees me." They showed me pictures, but none of the breasts really looked like my breasts, so I could never really translate it into how I thought I would look. Anyway, I'm happy with the result.

They put in a tissue expander during the mastectomy and injected it with saline periodically over several months until it was the right size. Because the expander is bigger than the implant will be, the skin feels tight. By the end, I was like, "Just get this thing out!" At three months when they do the last expansion, get a date to get the permanent implant put in, because otherwise what will happen is what happened to me—you wait too long.

I had no sensation in the tissue after I had the mastectomy. I have this huge scar and no feeling in the whole breast and surrounding tissue. So if it sounds grisly to have the tissue expander pulled out for the saline implant, it's really not, because you have no pain, so that's the good news. The surgeon went right back through the same scar, and although it wasn't exactly painful, it was just such a big deal that I felt incapacitated, couldn't use my right arm, couldn't exercise—the whole experience all over again.

After the nipple surgery, it's really gratifying, because the breast *looks* good. Before that, without the nipple it looked like an artificial breast. Really, you kind of think, "Why am I doing this? This looks so ridiculous, and the nipple's going to look really ridiculous." But it actually looks really good. For the nipple my surgeon used chest muscle—she pulled it up through—and for the aureole she went up under my arm and took muscle tissue from there, so I ended up with *another* scar. After that there's the tattoo to give it color— that's not a problem because there's no feeling.

Reconstruction is so hard. But it's all worth it.

Earlene's Story

Before I had surgery I had an opportunity to meet with my surgeon who examined me and advised a lumpectomy, given the size and location of the tumor. He and his nurse were available to answer questions. They also scheduled a preadmission routine at the hospital, which involved several hours at the hospital two days before my surgery. At that time a nurse specializing in cancer met with me and explained many of the details of what would be happening. She readily acknowledged that she knew that I must feel like I was on an "emotional roller coaster." She explained I would have the surgery and probably be able to go home within 24 hours, but that I would still have a surgical drain. I was encouraged to ask questions, and she assured me that she would either come to see me in the hospital or call after I went home to see how I was doing—which she did.

Don and I arrived at the hospital early the morning of my surgery, and he was able to stay with me until I was taken to the operating room. I was able to go directly to a small room where I changed into a hospital gown. I was given some special long socks to help prevent blood clots in my legs, and the nurse covered me in warmed blankets. A hospital bracelet was put around my wrist, and the nurse started an I.V.

The anesthesiologist came in and gave me some medication to help relax me. Don gave me a kiss and that was the last I remember before waking up in the recovery room.

Sometimes a fear comes as a surprise. At about ten o'clock at night, my husband had gone home and I couldn't get to sleep. In tears I explained to the nurse how afraid I was of being awake in the night terrified of the cancer and of what the lymph nodes would show. The nurse (Florence Nightingale reincarnated) came over to my bed, put her arm around my shoulder, gave me a hug, and said that we would figure out some way for me to get what I needed. The night shift nurse

(Florence Nightingale II) came in with jello and tea at two A.M. when I was awake and hungry, and she gave me another sleeping pill. I slept only about three hours that night, but I was not terrified.

I wasn't interested in anything but going home as soon as possible. Slowly but surely the contraptions were removed; a physical therapist demonstrated the exercises I was to do at home and gave me written instructions describing them. The surgeon saw me and gave me postoperative instructions. I got a ride in a wheelchair to the front door of the hospital where Don had the car waiting. Although I still continued to cry and worry if the cancer was in the lymph nodes, there was an enormous relief knowing that the tumor was gone.

Joann's Story

Some things have changed for the better. I had preadmission lab tests at the hospital, but did not see a cancer nurse. After my surgery I was told how to manage the drain at home. At the hospital I was given no information about support groups, nor did I see a physical therapist. I asked my surgeon about having physical therapy, but he said it wasn't necessary; however, after my radiation and chemotherapy treatments were over, my arm, chest, and back muscles got more and more stiff even though I seemed to be moving normally. Nine months after surgery I asked my oncologist about physical therapy, and she sent me right away; I wish I had insisted on it earlier. I still do these exercises and more, and I know I will need to do them all my life in order to have good strength and flexibility in my shoulder and arm. It is easy to let this go, and it is important not to.

I chose to have a lumpectomy, because in my case there would be no follow-up treatment difference between that and mastectomy. My surgery seemed so simple I was amazed. I went in early the morning of surgery. While I waited to be taken to the operating room Steve and I talked, and I spent some time meditating. I wasn't too afraid at that point—I just wanted that cancer out. I had wanted a local anesthetic used for the surgery, but was told that couldn't be done because of the location of the nerves involved; I had also asked for no preanesthesia medication, which *was* done. Meditating helped keep me calm and my blood pressure low. After the surgery, I had no nausea and almost no pain; I had only one three-inch incision. Because we already strongly suspected I had lymph node involvement, it was a relief to learn that only two nodes were positive. In spite of the advice we give about visitors, I felt pretty well, and I loved having one son bring his good friend to see me in the hospital. When I went home, my spirits were good—I was on the road to recovery.

✓ Checklist

- ❏ Organize things to take to the hospital.
- ❏ Don't take what you don't need.
- ❏ Discourage visits from friends while you're hospitalized.
- ❏ Arrange someone to take you to the hospital who will be there during surgery and notify family about how the surgery went.
- ❏ Make a list of what scares you—talk about these things with your physician.
- ❏ See a physical therapist before you leave the hospital—insist on it!

chapter 7

After Surgery—
and Before
Anything Else

The surgery is over and one of the steps toward recovery has
been taken. In contrast to the time spent in the hospital, when
you get home you will be able to decide what happens to you.
We can describe some of the steps we took to aid our recovery.
Everyone's personal treatment plan will look different, and the
plan will change depending on the stage of treatment you are in
at the moment. Generally there is not much time between
surgery and the beginning of any further treatment such as
chemotherapy and/or radiation therapy—usually just a couple of
weeks at most.

The Pathologist's Report

During that couple of weeks you will find out from your surgeon,
or your medical oncologist if you have one, the results of the
lymph node dissection. The pathologist will note how large the
tumor was and whether the cells it contained were duct cells or

lobular cells. The doctor will also comment on the margins. When the margins are clean, which means they do not contain any cancer cells, we know that the surgeon got all of the tumor. If the margins are not clean, then you would probably want to consider going to surgery again to make sure to get out the rest of the tumor. In the case of a larger tumor, some oncologists recommend having chemotherapy before surgery in order to reduce the size of the tumor and increase the likelihood of clean margins.

These latest pathology tests also give information about the general nature of the tumor; for example, how abnormal the cells look and how aggressive they appear to be—that is, whether or not they seem to be multiplying rapidly. The pathologist will also note whether the tumor is hormone receptor–positive, which means the growth of the tumor is promoted by either estrogen or progesterone hormones.

When pathologists turn their attention to the lymph nodes, they will note how many lymph nodes were retrieved during the surgery and whether any of them show cancer cells. Obviously, the higher the number of cancer-free lymph nodes the better. Remember, however, that whatever is found, there are treatments available. Having cancer cells in the lymph nodes is not a death sentence. Your oncologist will use all of the pathologist's report to make the best recommendation to you regarding treatment.

We will not go into any greater detail on the medical information, but we know that the pathology report will be on your mind. This is one of those times when there seems to be too much information to digest—and foreign information at that. For example, unless you are used to working in the metric system, you will probably not be able to readily translate the size of the tumor from centimeters into a more familiar measure. One centimeter is equal to about three-eighths of an inch. Your doctor should make some of these translations for you.

If the tumor is hormone receptor–positive, right away you may be starting treatment with tamoxifen, a medication that blocks growth-promoting effects of estrogen on the tumor. We have both taken tamoxifen, one pill twice a day. Joann had no side effects, Earlene had persistent hot flashes.

Lymphedema

Lymph is the tissue fluid passed through a series of filters called lymph nodes (see Figure 1.3, p. 6). Lymphedema means that lymph drainage is impaired, resulting in swelling (edema). This condition is caused by disturbance of the lymph system, such as that which occurs during the removal of nodes during breast surgery, and can affect the arm on that side. The swelling of the arm can be minor, or it can be extreme and disabling. Lymphedema can occur shortly after surgery or not until years later, so if you have had lymph nodes removed, you must be vigilant about the care of your arm for the rest of your life. Doctors believe that injury to the lymph system is the underlying cause of lymphedema, but no one understands why it happens to some patients and not to others, or why it might not show up for years following surgery. No one can even predict how many women who have had damage to the lymph nodes will develop lymphedema—a rough estimate is 10 to 30 percent.

Pain, concern about appearance, and limitation of movement make this an uncomfortable and sometimes embarrassing complication of having breast cancer. Unfortunately, once lymphedema is established, there is no permanent cure; however, there are many ways to manage it.

One of the best defenses against lymphedema is to take good care of your arm and avoid excessive strain or injury. **Do not let anyone take your blood pressure or draw blood from this arm.** Do not assume that a nurse or doctor will remember that you have had lymph node surgery on that side. Remind them. Earlene was hospitalized two years after her initial surgery, and she had big signs on her door and over her bed that said "DO NOT TAKE BLOOD PRESSURE OR DRAW BLOOD FROM RIGHT ARM." Get the same kind of signs if you ever have to be hospitalized.

Take good care of your skin, keeping it clean and moist and safe from injury. Wear a mitt when you take food out of the oven. Garden with gloves. If you get a hangnail, rub in some antibiotic cream. If you have **any** signs of infection, redness, or swelling in your arm or hand, call your doctor immediately. The more quickly an infection is treated, the less likely you are to have a permanent problem. Avoid excessive strain. Avoid carrying a heavy suitcase. Avoid extremes in heat and cold. Do eat well, rest well, and exercise—muscle contraction at healthy levels assists in lymph drainage.

Don't panic. Like everything else, in time it becomes second nature to be careful of your arm and hand. Some of you may have had breast cancer in both breasts and may have had lymph node removal on both sides, which makes care of both arms equally important and, we recognize, more difficult.

If you do develop lymphedema at some point, it is important to identify it early and get treatment as soon as possible. Your oncologist can refer you to specialists in the treatment of lymphedema. Many hospitals have specialized clinics and support groups for lymphedema patients. And insurance companies are now mandated by law to cover lymphedema treatment. Treatments include compression using special elastic "sleeves" (they look kind of like long gloves that fit the length of the arm); a specific kind of massage that assists lymph drainage; a specialized exercise program; and, in extreme cases, the use of a pump to help drain fluid. For more information, visit The National Lymphedema Network's web site at http://www.lymphnet.org/ or call 1-800-541-3259.

Constructing a Daily Treatment Plan

So, you are at home waiting for pathology results or for the next stage of treatment, and you need to have your own active treatment plan. One approach to the construction of a treatment plan is to make a daily plan—something you can do easily. A sample plan for the time immediately after surgery might go something like this:

Morning:

1. *Taking Care of the Drain:* Ask your helper to empty the Jackson-Pratt drain and record the amount, or you can do it yourself, if you prefer.

2. *The Problem of the Shower:* Tub baths are usually not allowed until after the drain is removed, and you may wonder what exactly to do with this extra appendage—the drain—during your shower. You can have both hands free in the shower by tying a cloth belt, such as the belt from your bathrobe, around your waist and pinning the drain to that. Nancy Floyd Turner, a breast cancer survivor, was so vexed by this problem that she designed the Marsupial Pouch, a terry cloth bag to hold your drain and other sundries while in the shower. If you want one, you can call Derma Sciences (1-800-825-4325). Once you are clean and dry, the drain can be pinned to the soft cotton bra we mentioned or to any other handy article of clothing. Cotton pads or cotton balls can be placed over the incision or under the insertion point of the drain for greater comfort. We found that the drain need not be obvious and is nicely hidden under loose-fitting clothing if you want to go out during the day. Using a blower to dry your hair may be difficult at first if your surgery has been on the side of your dominant hand, because it is generally uncomfortable to raise your arm on the side of the surgery. This is something a close friend can help you with.

3. *Breakfast:* Remember, good nutrition is important to help your body heal and to give you strength, so don't let pain, tiredness, or depression stop you from eating as normally and as healthfully as possible. If you aren't able to eat for any of these reasons, talk to your doctor about this.

4. *Mental Therapy:* Around breakfast time may be a time when you need to take pain medication—different people need differing amounts or kinds of medication. Earlene took some pain medication early in the morning and then meditated, which allowed time for the pain medication to work so she was comfortable while doing the physical therapy exercises. Listening to the tape, completing her exercises, seeing improvement all the time, and being pain-free helped create a positive outlook for the morning.

You may want to take some morning time for writing in a journal. You may want to talk with a friend instead. We found quiet time and reflection helpful. One form of quiet time is meditation. You can listen to tapes or meditate several times a day or at particularly stressful times. Joann had no need for pain medication; she usually had breakfast, then meditated in the early-morning sunlight for a half-hour or so before going on with her day. Throughout this process we both noticed an increase in the intensity of our awareness of life around us.

5. Physical Therapy: Before you were discharged from the hospital, you should have been seen by a physical therapist who has prescribed a few basic exercises. These are important to keep you from losing strength and flexibility in your arm and shoulder. If you were not told about any exercises, ask your surgeon if there is any reason you should not exercise. If there are no such reasons, we can give you a few exercises that might be helpful to you. Whatever you do, be gentle with yourself. Don't push yourself so hard that you hurt yourself, but it will be beneficial for you to do some exercise.

Stretching: For all of these exercises, begin slowly and hold any stretch for just a few seconds. Your goal should be to hold a position for 60 seconds, but **don't expect to be able to do that at first.** As with any exercise or stretch, if you feel pain—STOP—and consult your doctor or physical therapist. When you can, keep doing these stretches, maybe forever, because your underarm and shoulder can stiffen up even after years. They are good for everyone, even those who have never had breast surgery.

1. Lie on the floor on your back. Place your hands under your head with your elbows pointing toward the ceiling (Figure 7.1). Let your elbows drop toward the floor until you achieve a gentle stretch. Hold this for 30 seconds, then release and repeat for a total of 5 stretches.

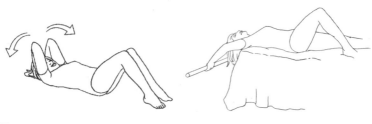

Figure 7.1   Figure 7.2

2. Lie on the floor on your back. With your arms outstretched in T formation, bend your elbows upward at a right angle. Gradually scoot your arms up as if to straighten them over your head. Let the floor support them and push them as far as you can without hurting yourself, gradually stretching them until after a few days you can pretty much straighten them out.

3. After you can do the first exercise, try the same exercise standing against a wall. This time you will have to push a little harder to reach up above your head because gravity is working against you.

4. Lie on the bed on your back with the top of your head at the side edge of the bed. With straight arms, lift a broomstick up over your chest and let the broomstick arch back over your head as in Exercise 1 (Figure 7.2). When you can reach all the way, the broomstick and your hands will be hanging out over the floor. Count to five. Then, keeping your arms straight, move the broomstick back above your chest and down. As the days go on, increase the count so that you are continuing to stretch your chest and underarm area.

5. Standing with your arms out to your sides, bend your elbows upward at a right angle, and grasp the sides of a doorway (Figure 7.3). Lean forward into the open doorway, stretching your chest area open. Hold for a few seconds. Increase this count a little each day, until you can hold this position for 60 seconds. Then you can begin to push a little farther into the doorway to increase the stretch.

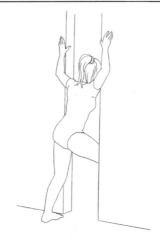

Figure 7.3

Strengthening: For any exercise you should work both sides, injured or not. This ensures that you will increase muscle strength evenly. Try to do everything in control and as smoothly as possible, not jerking anything into position or dropping out of position. A good goal might be two or three sets of ten repetitions, but as with the stretches, start slowly and build up to your goal. Again, it is important not to hurt yourself. After you can reach above your head, try these exercises:

1. Lie on your stomach, arms stretched above your head (Figure 7.4). Lift one hand as far as you can and then return it to the floor. Do five repetitions with each arm. If you want to increase, do more sets of five; then add one or two repetitions

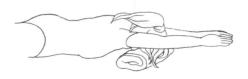

Figure 7.4

until this all becomes easy. Then you can add a little weight—not much—just hold something in your hand as you do the exercise. Cans from the kitchen make good beginning weights—you can start with 6 or 8 ounces and work up to 16 ounces, which is a pound. That's probably enough for this exercise.

2. Lie on your side in a comfortable position. Reach up toward the ceiling with your free hand (Figure 7.5). Make circles with your hand, varying the diameter of the circle. Then reverse the direction of the circle. As usual, start with a small number, working up to 15 or 20 revolutions each direction. Do this on the other side, too. When this becomes easy, you can add a little weight as in the first exercise; you can increase the weight, but you don't need to lift any more than a pound.

3. Lie on your back as you did for the stretching exercise with the broomstick. Push the broomstick up toward the ceiling, then lower it (Figure 7.6). This will probably be easy, so when you feel like it, you could put a couple of one-pound cans from the kitchen in each hand and push them to the ceiling. Try increasing the repetitions and number of sets, but don't hurt yourself. You're trying to make yourself feel better, not worse!

By the time you can do all of these exercises comfortably, you may want to invest in an exercise book to help you keep working on stretching and strengthening your arms and shoulders. A good one for stretching is *Sport Stretch,* by Michael J. Alter. Check out some exercise books from your local library so you

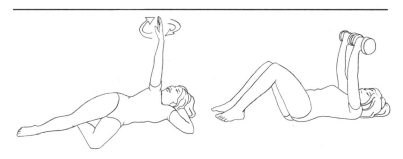

Figure 7.5   Figure 7.6

can find one that suits your needs—remember that you are trying to help your body, not enter a muscle woman contest. Another suggestion we have is that you incorporate a walk into your daily routine; it may be very short to begin with unless you are in the habit of taking walks, but it will be good for both your mental and physical health.

The Rest of the Day: The rest of the day will certainly be taken up with many of the usual things you might have done before surgery. We can't imagine anyone going back to work at least until the drain is removed, but each person has individual needs around this issue. We imagine that there are more people out there saying that they went back to work too soon rather than that they stayed away too long. There are a few things that may just be too much of a pain—literally—like ironing. You probably won't feel like cooking every night—there were weeks where neither of us cooked—there may even be months when you won't, either.

1. Rest: Getting enough rest is an important ingredient for healing. Your nighttime sleep may be interrupted for a number of reasons. You may have discomfort from the surgery, you may be awakened by hot flashes, or you may awaken because of anxiety or depression. If you are not sleeping well at night, you might want to try napping, or, alternatively, using the meditative position called *savasana,* in which you lie on the floor, either with your legs extended and feet slightly apart or with your knees bent and falling together, your arms extended somewhat away from your body, palms up. When you meditate in this position, you can rest your body and mind even though you are not sleeping. Cover yourself with a light blanket if you like. Even fifteen minutes will refresh you. If you fall asleep, that's okay—you probably needed it more than you knew. A warm shower or a back rub may help. Avoiding caffeine and alcohol will certainly help, and if all of these suggestions fail, you should ask your doctor for medication to help with this problem.

2. Other Helpful Ingredients to Recovery: As you look into breast cancer treatments, you will find a number of alternative therapies that are available. We don't believe in abandoning traditional medical treatments in favor of any alternatives, but we do believe additional therapies can complement your treatment. Keep in mind these are unlikely to be paid for by your insurance, but you can ask your company if it does cover any of these. We found deep tissue massage, weekly if possible, to be very therapeutic, both physically and emotionally. (We learned that a prescription from a doctor for "neuromuscular" massage, which is the deep tissue kind, will be enough to get some insurance companies to pay for it.) Some other alternatives might be acupuncture or hypnotherapy. Whatever you do to increase your sense of well being can only be good for you.

A support group may provide the kind of personal understanding that is especially helpful. In Chapter 1 we encouraged you to look into taking part in a support group, especially one for newly diagnosed breast cancer patients. An educational group is another helpful kind of group to look for. If you have trouble finding a group that meets your needs and you feel comfortable going to, look for another. However, don't let yourself get upset if you can't find a good support group—if you have the positive, constant support of friends or family, you will get along fine.

Psychotherapy, either weekly or more or less often, can also provide a place where you can voice your feelings and concerns. All of us go into our illness with a unique personal history that colors our experience of the illness. Psychotherapy can help you make the most of your treatment, help you avoid a "victim" role, and help you construct the most positive and helpful treatment plan for yourself. In addition, if you are depressed, whether from the stresses that go along with having cancer or from side effects of treatments, a good therapist will recognize whether or not you need medication.

For more ideas on constructing a daily self-treatment plan, read Chapter 6 of *The Alpha Book on Cancer & Living* (1993). Alameda, Calif.: The Alpha Institute, especially pages 211–231.

Special Circumstances

Our hearts go out particularly to women with young children. Our children were adults when we were diagnosed, and neither of us had to do any more than take care of ourselves. Since women are having children later in life, we are sure more and more women diagnosed with breast cancer will have small children, and this situation requires special planning and creativity.

Other special circumstances may involve having to care for someone else, such as an ill spouse or an aging parent. We recognize that there are many different circumstances requiring all kinds of resourcefulness. In general, the more people who depend on you, the more you will have to ask for help from others to get everything done. When you are a caregiver for others, the best thing you can do for them is to help yourself first. Your physician or the hospital social worker can help you find resources to help care for those who depend on you. We hope that you will use the idea of creating your own treatment plan to help you cope with the special problems of your life.

❑   ❑   ❑

Earlene's Story

After I found I was incinerating articles of clothing, I went to see a psychiatrist skilled in treating patients with medical illness. Explaining to me how I was building a new relationship with myself was one of the many ways he helped me. "What do you have to do when you build a new relationship?" he asked. Then while I listened he answered gently, "The first thing you have to do is show up. You won't get anywhere if you don't show up for yourself."

This meant that I needed to construct my care plan and then I had to show up—become dependable and reliable about taking good care of myself. My plan, which included a short daily walk, meditation, physical therapy exercises, and writing in my journal, brought a pleasant rhythm to my day in an otherwise miserable time. Don't forget to include massage if you can.

Joann's Story

Although at first I was meditating every day, using a subliminal healing tape, I really didn't take very good care of myself. A few days after surgery I went on a week-long trip to visit family; then I began radiation treatment, at 3:30 every weekday, and I had my first chemotherapy treatment the same day that I went in to begin my preparations for the new school year. I tried to cut everything at work to the essentials so I could leave each day in time for radiation. I didn't exercise; I started to skip morning meditation—got it in, maybe, at the end of the afternoon. All of this was a recipe for disaster, and I was able to keep this pace for less than six weeks, at which time my body said, "Enough! Stop!" and put me in the hospital. Then I took leave of absence for three months. During that leave, I learned to follow some of the advice we've included in this chapter.

✓ Checklist

❑ Take your tape recorder when you hear the pathologist's report and when you are given treatment options.

❑ Construct a daily treatment plan:

Rest

Take care of surgical problems

Nutrition

Mental therapy

Meditation

Support group/person

Physical therapy

Exercise

Massage

❑ Arrange for child-care relief.

❑ Arrange for household help.

chapter 8

Radiation

Radiation (or X-ray) therapy is a fairly standard component of treatment for many kinds of cancer, including breast cancer. In times past it was not possible to regulate radiation doses well; this resulted in burns and other kinds of radiation damage. Consequently, some people think they should avoid radiation at all cost. Today, a dosimetrist calculates the precise amount of radiation a patient will receive, and highly skilled technicians plan the placement of the rays, monitor blood counts, and deliver the therapy under the close supervision of a radiation oncologist who is part of the staff of a hospital or special clinic where you are likely to go for treatment. Radiation therapy usually requires a treatment every day, Monday through Friday, for six to seven weeks. When you are referred for radiation therapy, choose a hospital that treats many people. As with other medical procedures, the more procedures a hospital staff does, the better off you will be in their hands.

What You May Experience

The first visit with a radiation oncologist will be shortly after whatever surgery you have had, based on your surgeon's or oncologist's recommendations for further treatment. The radiation oncologist will review your pathology and surgery reports and plan whatever radiation therapy is appropriate in

your case. The doctor should introduce you to the nurses and
technicians in the unit, who should acquaint you with the
equipment to be used, the dressing rooms, and the procedures
used in their waiting rooms.

At this appointment the physician may give you some
pamphlets about their procedures. If it isn't included, one
pamphlet you should get from the American Cancer Society is
Radiation Therapy and You, by calling 1-800-ACS-2345. Take the
time to read this carefully along with any other reading material
the radiation oncologist gives you. Call the doctor with any
questions you have. If during this appointment you don't feel you
have adequate control of your treatment, or you don't have your
fears and questions addressed, ask your surgeon or primary care
doctor for a referral to another physician or hospital. This is
another time to find medical helpers you trust. When you are
comfortable with what you are being told, you can proceed with
such matters as signing consent forms, arranging a time in your
schedule, often daily, when you can arrive at the hospital for
treatment.

The Simulation

Probably the second experience you will have with radiation
therapy will be a long (two hours or more) appointment during
which the technicians set up the exact areas where you will
receive the radiation. During this time the technicians will map
out the exact area over your breast that will receive radiation to
make sure you receive radiation only where it is needed and
make sure that nearby tissue, such as your lungs, are not
exposed. It is important for you to have someone with you,
someone you are okay about seeing your recently scarred and
damaged chest, someone who will speak up for you if things
don't go the way you want, someone who can get whatever you
need. Take that person *into the room* with you—no radiation will
be given that day, and it isn't enough to have that person in the
waiting room. You are still vulnerable, and this long and stressful

session can be hard to cope with. In this setting the technicians expect you to be as still as possible, not talking or moving. Both of us found ourselves seriously emotionally violated by events that occurred during this procedure, and because we were alone, we had no one to help us.

The room where the simulation takes place is darkened, and thin beams of light are focused on your chest wall and breast. The technician(s) will probably draw various configurations on your skin with markers. These marks will wash away in a couple of days. What look like television monitors are mounted to the wall upon which you can see lots of numbers flash by. The technician is typically intent on making sure your body is in the right position and will be busy with equipment and calculations.

1. Pictures: During this session, the technicians will probably want to take your picture. One kind will be of your face; this is to identify you when you come for therapy and ensure that the technicians have **your** file when they set up for you. Another kind will be of the breast area they intend to radiate. These photos are Polaroids, and you should ask to see them and make sure they are acceptable to you. We are not saying they should be beautiful photographs—just make sure they are not taken when you are in tears or they are not grotesque pictures of your breast that include your face. The technicians should respect your feelings and your right to privacy.

2. Cradle: You will be asked to spend a long period of time with your arm extended above your head, placed in what is referred to as a "cradle." It is neither a comfortable nor a comforting apparatus. If you have been doing some stretching exercises since your surgery, this will be easier for you. During the simulation the technicians are working to find the exact position you need, and this takes time. Each day when you have radiation therapy, the technicians will position your arm in the cradle; however, the actual therapy takes only a few minutes. Before they begin, ask if there will be any time you can have a break or if you can move when the technicians are not working with you. Ask them to tell you what they will be doing as the procedure goes along and why. Ask them to let you know how long you will need to hold a position. There may be times when the technicians are in the middle of a complicated measurement or calculation and they may need to postpone answering, but they should be courteous about it. Sometimes, to make the procedure more comfortable, you can listen to a radio or to tapes. However, it is important that you not move unexpectedly since that may prolong an already tiring experience.

3. Plaster Mold: One of the last procedures the technician may complete during the mock session is making a plaster contour molding of the breast. This is not uncomfortable, but by the time they do it, you will probably be ready to be done.

4. Tattoos: In the pamphlets and literature you receive, there might be references to "semipermanent" tattoos. Tattoos are routinely used to make aligning the X-ray equipment easier for the technicians; the *marks* are important and necessary for your treatment. It is not clear to us, however, what a "semipermanent" tattoo is. A tattoo is an indelible mark made by inserting pigment under the skin or by the production of scars. The procedure is not painless, and it is permanent. The technicians like them because they *are* permanent. They are tiny, barely perceptible dots on your neck and/or chest, and the number required may vary from two or three to several. If you are not bothered by this, you will find it simple to have the tattoos, and the technicians will want to do this during the simulation. If you do not want tattoos, there are options. Discuss this with the radiation oncologist beforehand, because the technicians are likely to insist that you must have them, but that is not the case. If you decide to have the tattoos and later wish to have them removed, that can be done by laser, but your insurance probably will not cover that procedure. If you do not want tattoos, it is possible for the technicians to re-mark you daily—or you can learn to replace the marks yourself—with a permanent marker if you are careful not to wash these marks totally away. This is your body; you choose what works best for you.

Treatment

You will be asked to put on a hospital gown and lie down on the X-ray table in a larger, cool room where there may be what look like television monitors around the room that display computer information to the technicians. The gown will be removed from the breast to be treated. The table is similar to the one you experienced during the simulation, and the X-ray equipment should look familiar, too. It is a huge machine with a rotating arm—sometimes technicians will make an effort to brighten this for patients, such as by taping pictures of flowers on the arm so that when it is over them patients can see the pictures, but often they do not.

The technician will position you in the cradle, lying on your back. The process of being irradiated takes only a few minutes, even if the technician has to do more than one angle. The technician will leave the room and you will be required to lie very still while you hear the buzzing noise of the machine. Unlike having a chest X-ray, you can breathe normally during these times, because they can last more than a minute each, and the technicians may need to place the machine in more than one position.

Before the first treatment you will probably have an opportunity to negotiate the time of your daily treatments. If you are working or caring for children, it may be especially helpful to schedule your treatment at a particular time of the day. Other considerations could be important to you, such as completing your self-care program before having a treatment later in the morning. Neither of us had a problem scheduling these treatments at a daily time convenient for us.

The technician will check your skin frequently for any changes, especially as your treatment progresses. Once a week Earlene's appointments were longer because several extra tasks had to be accomplished. She was weighed and two extra X-rays were taken to recheck the exact positioning of the treatments. In addition, she met with the radiation oncologist who examined the skin and reviewed the progress of the treatment. The length of your radiation therapy depends on the total desired dose of radiation having been delivered over a period of time. Our treatments were six and seven weeks; the number of treatment days required to deliver this total dose can vary among patients.

During these weeks your blood will be monitored to be sure your white blood cell count does not drop below a certain limit. If you are not routinely seeing a medical oncologist, blood counts may be done as part of the review of the progress of your treatment. If you have to have chemotherapy at the same time, there are plenty of opportunities to get the information needed without additional blood draws. You do get to the point, pretty quickly, where you don't want any more needle sticks than are absolutely essential.

Caring for Your Skin

Soft cotton bras, no underwires, maybe a T-shirt instead.

Aloe vera gel, no deodorants (see the advice in Chapter 4).

Saltwater soaks can be soothing to the skin. Dissolve one teaspoon of salt in a quart of warm water. Saturate a wash cloth or soft dish towel with the solution and apply to the radiated area 3 or 4 times a day. Apply Vanicream (or other cream approved by your radiation oncologist) following the soaks.

No creams, "natural" or otherwise that might contain estrogen, unless your tumor is not receptor-positive. Vitamin E creams or cocoa butter are great. (Have you ever wanted to smell like a giant chocolate bar? Now's your chance.)

If you choose to re-mark yourself daily, ask the technicians how to do it; in addition, you will need to be careful when you bathe not to scrub away the previous day's marks. After your bath, mark them again so they can't fully disappear.

Watch both your chest and back for any signs of radiation burns. Your chest area will become somewhat tanned-looking, which is usually not a problem. If you develop overly dry, flaky, itchy, or red patches, alert the technician right away, and treat these areas as prescribed.

While you are having radiation treatment (and even afterward), you should protect your skin from the sun. Cover the treatment area fully with clothing (don't forget your neck area). Since burning is already a risk, you need to take every precaution to keep from having any additional burns. Right now, not even titanium dioxide or zinc oxide sun blocks are good enough.

How You Will Feel

Except for the discomfort of the cradle, the coolness of the room, the hardness of the table, physically, radiation treatment itself is easy. You may go through the entire procedure with few side effects. Some people don't feel a lot of tiredness, but don't be surprised if it creeps up on you. The effects of radiation build up over a period of time, and at first you will probably not notice any difference. As the days go by, however, you may feel increasingly tired, and by the end of treatment become exhausted. It will help to get plenty of rest, to eat healthfully, and to take good care of your skin.

Psychologically, radiation can seem a relief in comparison with other treatments you may have had or may yet face. It becomes a predictable ritual, and this predictability can be somewhat comforting. Often radiation units are generally warm and inviting with a pot of hot water always on for a cup of tea or cocoa and a candy jar on the reception counter. The reception staff always has a smile. When you go somewhere every day for weeks and weeks, you get to know the staff, and they you, and there is comfort in nodding and smiling to the patient just before you and just after.

That's the good news. The other side is that it can be just as psychologically challenging as other treatments. Every day you must lie down and receive your treatment in a room where no one else can enter.

Sometimes patients don't realize how tired they are becoming toward the end of radiation treatment. Although you may think it is nothing to drive yourself to treatments, it might be helpful to have some alternatives in mind. If it's convenient, taking the daily trip to and from the hospital on the bus, subway, or train could provide some much-needed time for resting or meditating.

In addition to the fatigue, the breast tissue will likely become somewhat swollen and tender. It can take many months, even more than a year for this to resolve. Although this side effect is generally not a problem, we could think of two instances where it is: getting a very vigorous hug and when you go for your first postradiation mammogram. Be sure to tell the mammographer that you have had surgery and radiation and that your breast is still tender so that she will be extra gentle with you.

❑   ❑   ❑

Earlene's Story

I don't want to remember the simulation day when I ended up with tattoos against my wishes and photographs that should not have included my face. I felt so terrible and humiliated. I tried to explain my concerns and feelings to the technician, but she was truly clueless. I guess one clueless individual in three months of treatment is not so bad, but it really felt awful at the time. Fortunately, my radiation oncologist was very understanding and made sure that the tattoos were removed by laser after my treatments were complete, and she had my face cut out of the photographs. This experience was so unlike the rest of my days at this unit where everyone was so warm and concerned.

I remember some weeks into the treatment, lying on the radiation table thinking that instead of crying I could use some imagery to help me through. When the radiation was administered, the machine emitted a buzzing sound. Each time I heard this sound I would imagine cancer cells frying—sizzling and curling up and dying. I liked that picture and felt more in control.

I also remember warmly those days my husband or son drove me to the treatments. If I wasn't too tired afterward, we would stop for coffee or lunch. It was so comforting to have company.

Joann's Story

I still have not totally gotten rid of my anger over what happened at my simulation session. That day would be easy, I thought—just a simulation, no radiation—so I went alone, which was a terrible mistake. The technicians explained nothing about what they were doing, talked to each other as though I were not even there, and left me alone in the cold room, bare-breasted, with my arm over my head for more than half an hour, without explanation or apology. I'll never know where I found the strength to insist my way out of tattoos and refuse photographs of my swollen, weeping face. I had experienced $2\frac{1}{2}$ hours of pain, abandonment, and debasement, and ended up sobbing over the steering wheel of my car in the parking lot. No one should underestimate how vulnerable you are or how anxious you are to be a perfect patient in order to get well; no one can predict how a certain situation will affect you.

There is a bottom line: All the staff has to do is to explain exactly what they want to do before they start, to tell you how long it will take, and to listen to what you have to say. Especially, they shouldn't leave you alone. That doesn't sound too complicated, does it?

✓ Checklist

❏ Take someone with you and into all preradiation visits.

❏ Insist that every step be explained.

❏ Let technicians know if you are tired and what you need.

❏ Gather products to use in caring for your skin—and use them faithfully.

❏ Watch your skin carefully for burns or other changes.

❏ Follow your daily treatment plan.

❏ Get information about alternatives to driving to radiation treatments.

chapter 9

Chemotherapy

We have already recommended that you seek help from an oncologist soon after your diagnosis so you have someone coordinating your cancer treatment even though you may not need chemotherapy. If the node dissection or other factors indicate you may need chemotherapy and you haven't already seen an oncologist, your surgeon will send you to one at this point. The oncologist should describe fully the length of your treatment, the drug or combination of drugs to be used, how and when they will be administered, and all of their possible side effects. This is another time when you will need your tape recorder, a note pad, and another set of ears. Our oncologist gave out all of this information in writing in addition to her verbal explanation.

The two ways to receive chemotherapy for breast cancer are (1) oral or (2) intravenous (I.V.). You should be shown the treatment rooms; often chemotherapy is given in the doctor's office, but sometimes it can be done at home or must be given in the hospital. If you need to be hospitalized for chemotherapy treatments, you should be told why, how long you will be in the hospital, and how the treatment is done. You should be given a chance to ask every question you have.

Choosing an oncologist is an extremely important step in your treatment. You are giving this person enormous power over your life, and you will be seeing this doctor for several years after your treatment has finished. You must be able to have utmost trust in your oncologist, you must be able to confide fully, you must be able to feel listened to, you must feel cared about as a human being. Relating to a physician in this way may be difficult if you have not had many experiences with a doctor. You have to take the time to choose carefully. It is not medically imperative for you to begin chemotherapy or any other treatment instantly. If you are dissatisfied with the way you are spoken to, with feeling rushed through an appointment, with the way your questions are answered (or not answered), with the way the office staff handles your phone calls and waiting room time, or even with the treatment proposed for you, discuss these concerns with the oncologist and/or ask your surgeon or primary care physician for other referrals.

When you have been diagnosed with cancer, sometimes fear of the treatments you may have to undergo can be nearly as great as the fear of death. Many of us have heard terrible tales of side effects of chemotherapy—hair loss, nausea, sores in the mouth, exhaustion—that serve to fuel that fear unnecessarily. We do not intend to minimize the difficulty of undergoing chemotherapy for breast cancer; however, we want to reassure you that side effects are manageable and treatable, and there are things you can do to make this part of your treatment easier.

1. Devise a daily self-care plan. Take care of your physical and emotional needs *every day.* This can be similar, if not identical, to the plan you created after your surgery—if you are having chemotherapy before you have surgery, look at our suggestions in Chapter 7. Set aside a time to meditate once or even twice a day. Make yourself exercise, even if you only walk to the end of your driveway and back. Be sure to pamper yourself: warm baths help; try some aromatherapy; have a massage, weekly if you can afford it. Write in a journal daily, even if you destroy it later; it can help to name your fears and feelings. Write about how you feel physically—this may be helpful if you need to recall symptoms for your physician.

2. Report any and all discomforts, problems, and questions to your physician. Your doctor will want to know what you need help with, and it is comforting to know that side effects such as nausea and teary eyes can be controlled. If your energy level seems extremely low you may have low blood counts, and medications are available to keep this from happening. Most important, report at once any fever (if you don't feel well, remember to take your temperature), which may be a sign of infection.

3. Save your veins. Ask about having a port. A port is a catheter that is put into a vein (often beneath the collarbone) and usually remains in place until you have completed all of your chemotherapy treatments to facilitate both administering chemotherapy and drawing blood for the many tests that need to be done to monitor you. If you experience problems with having I.V. delivery of the chemotherapy drugs, ask right away about having a port. Some chemotherapy drugs can't be given safely without a port, and in that case your oncologist will tell you one is necessary to facilitate your treatment. A port needs some special care, and that should be described to you before you decide on one. After chemotherapy is over, the port is removed.

If you do not need or want a port, you can still reserve your veins for chemotherapy. Hospital labs usually want to draw a vial of blood from your arm, when all they really need is just a few drops in a thin tube for a blood count. This blood can be collected by a simple poke of a finger. If you would rather have a finger stick, just ask for it. They may have to come back to get your blood later because they don't have the equipment with them. That's okay—tell them to come back.

4. Visit the dentist before you begin treatment. You will probably be undergoing treatment for several months, so if you have not seen your dentist for a while, the time to do this is before you begin treatment. During chemotherapy treatment for cancer, several oral problems, such as mouth sores, bleeding, or increased incidence of infection, can arise that will make it inadvisable for you to have dental work done. This said, don't hesitate to go during treatment if you have a dental emergency. If an emergency arises, ask your oncologist if there is anything special your dentist should do, and be sure to advise your dentist that you are undergoing chemotherapy treatment for cancer.

5. Hair considerations. When hair is damaged by chemotherapy, it can thin dramatically or fall out altogether. Don't be shocked if you lose other hair, such as eyelashes or pubic hair. Don't perm or color your hair before (or for a while after) undergoing chemotherapy, because the chemicals used on your hair are damaging, and the chemo will be, too. Well-meaning friends may suggest icing your scalp or using vitamin or other treatments to keep your hair from falling out. Don't ice your scalp unless you have clearance from your doctor. The other treatments probably won't help and just cost money. Do keep your hair nicely trimmed and styled; some people even want to shave it all off rather than lose it in clumps. As we suggested earlier, if you think you might want to wear a wig, pick it out before treatment begins so you can choose one that matches your own hair (unless of course you've always wanted to be a blonde—give it a whirl!). Some people may be disturbed by the lack of eyebrows and eyelashes in contrast to the fullness of a wig; a makeup professional can help you with this, or you can opt for turbans and scarves.

What You May Experience

Many people have heard about side effects of chemotherapy: nausea, exhaustion, hair loss, and so on. When talking to you about possible side effects, the doctor tries to cover everything, and you should be informed about long-term or delayed risks of chemotherapy, such as infertility, menopause, heart problems, or secondary cancers. Some effects aren't mentioned, probably because they don't cause anything terribly debilitating. We think you might want to know about them, though.

One side effect of chemotherapy is common enough to have a pet name. "Chemo brain" is disconcerting and a nuisance, and although it is worst during treatment, it can last for years in some form or another. This phenomenon may make you think you are becoming senile, because it causes memory blanks. These blanks can be scary; for example, if you forget you've made a phone call and then turn around and a few minutes later make it again, having the same discussion with the person you've called, that person can become alarmed, understandably. It will be alarming to you, too, to find out you've done that, but unless this becomes a huge problem for you, don't dwell on it. The most common complaint we've heard is "losing" words in the middle of a sentence, even words you use routinely. They are just not there when you want to say them; however, they're only temporarily missing and will be available when you want them next.

A possible side effect of the Ativan used to prevent or treat nausea is amnesia, which may last from four to six hours. Our oncologist tells of patients who failed to remember watching videos right after receiving chemotherapy; if you are aware that Ativan can cause such memory lapses, you may choose not to take it.

Some people experience soreness on the scalp that feels like their hair roots are hurting. Of course, hair roots themselves have no nerve cells—you know it doesn't hurt when your hair falls out—but this feels so specific that's what you think is happening. This soreness doesn't mean your hair is falling out or that you will lose your hair.

Because chemotherapy affects the cells that grow most quickly, such as hair and nails (and cancer cells), you will probably see changes in your nails as well as in your hair. Sometimes fingernails become dry and brittle; other times they can actually become less so. The oddest change may be in your toenails, which may blacken as though they've been hit with a hammer. This may occur because the pressure of shoes (especially if they fit tightly) causes a little bleeding to occur under those nails.

During chemotherapy you will have a tendency to bleed a bit more easily—bumping your leg on the dishwasher door may cause more severe damage than you'd usually have. Keep a supply of bandaids handy.

Certain drugs used may cause a metallic taste in your mouth, which can come and go or be very persistent. This may cause some foods to become less appealing to you. You might get relief by chewing gum, such as the new baking soda–based chewing gums, or by sucking on lemon drops. Don't use mouthwashes to try to get rid of this—they won't help much, because this problem is in your system. Also, many mouthwashes contain alcohol, which can irritate already sensitive oral tissues.

It is not unusual for chemo patients to experience weight gain. You may think that couldn't be possible because food can be terribly unappealing at times. However, the medications themselves cause the weight gain, and there is not much you can do about this. It is not in your best interest to be dieting during this time, because you need nourishment. It *is* in your best interest to select healthful, fresh foods to eat, such as vegetables and fruits and other foods low in fat and sugars. Try to eat for your good health rather than to eat for your psychological comfort, which may result in your overindulging in less healthful foods. Foods high in fat and sugars can contribute to stomach upsets.

Some chemotherapy drugs are dreadfully hard on the bladder; you will be instructed to drink certain amounts of water and empty your bladder frequently in the hours immediately after a treatment. This should be your standard all the time. Be sure to keep your doctor informed about urinary problems of any kind.

For some women sexual intercourse can cause urinary tract irritations and/or infections under ordinary circumstances. In such cases, intercourse during chemotherapy may be especially problematic because of increased bladder sensitivity. Discuss sexual concerns with your partner—disinterest in or discomfort during intercourse does not preclude other kinds of intimacy. If you experience a troublesome loss of libido that carries over into the posttreatment period, speak with your doctor about whether this might be caused by estrogen or testosterone deficiency and what might help you.

Some of the notorious side effects may not be as well controlled as you hope. Nausea is one. If you have persistent nausea, your doctor can try different medications to help with this problem. Mouth sores can be awful, causing eating and oral hygiene problems. Again, some medications are helpful to a degree, but you may not be able to get a lot of relief—avoid mouthwashes and acidic or hard foods; you can brush your teeth with your finger or a soft washcloth or use a baking soda mouthwash if necessary. Fluorouracil and other chemotherapies cause teary eyes; this, too, can be alleviated somewhat by eyedrops, but perhaps not entirely.

Things to Take with You

- *A good friend.* Someone will need to take you to and from your chemotherapy treatments, because you should not drive afterward. Unless it is completely unavoidable, it is not good enough to be dropped off and picked up. You need to take your friend into the treatment room with you to hold your hand and reassure you that you are not alone. You may not feel talkative. That's okay—it is not your job to entertain anyone. Ask your friend to stay with you at home afterward. You might need help, and this is not a time to be alone. This is just our opinion—we have heard of folks who do not want anyone with them during their treatments, even going to the extreme of arriving and being picked up by taxi. This is hard for us to imagine, because we were so dependent on our family and friends, and it is not what we recommend, but we respect your need to do whatever fits you.

- *A cassette or CD player with earphones.* Take something soothing to play during your treatment: gentle music is good, as are visualization and meditation tapes. Choose something calming. Visualizing your treatment attacking and killing those weak, deformed cancer cells will be more helpful to you than feeling poisoned.

- *A talisman.* Any symbol of your spiritual strength will remind you to access that strength whenever you need it.

❑   ❑   ❑

Joann's Story

I hated chemotherapy, resisted it the whole way, begged every time not to have to go, and counted down to the end. For six months I was sick and found nothing good about any of it. My husband sat beside me and visualized bubbles of good, healing stuff dripping in, but I knew I was being poisoned; but really, deep down I believed what was being poisoned was the cancer and that I would be cured.

What was the treatment like? My treatment schedule was two weeks of chemotherapy followed by two weeks of recovery. I was given a combination of drugs administered I.V. A tablet dissolved under my tongue helped me relax quickly while the nurse inserted a butterfly needle into a vein somewhere on my hand or arm—it was a different place each time. Finally I talked to my doctor about having a port, and she was willing, but by that time I was more than halfway through and decided not to bother.

During the treatment I became sleepy and disoriented. For the first few moments as they went in, some of the drugs felt cold and some burned, but those feelings didn't last long; because I had trouble accepting the treatment, my mind may have made them seem worse than they actually were. After about an hour, Steve would tell me there wasn't much left, and he would count down as the last drops left the line and went into my arm.

I had some side effects: After each of my treatments, my scalp hurt, I ached all over like I had the flu; I lost my toenails (but not my fingernails); the tears in my eyes at my son's college graduation ceremonies were from 5 FU; the sores in my mouth kept me from eating a friend's 25th anniversary dinner; most of my hair fell out, including my eyelashes and much of my body hair. I didn't even need to shave my legs. I thought if chemo did this to my good cells, the weaker, bad ones were surely dead.

Very scary times for me during my treatment came when I was hospitalized two times in three weeks—first for pericarditis (an inflammation of the membrane surrounding the heart) and second for systemic infection two weeks later—and I began a three-month leave of absence from work with the first hospitalization. The symptoms of pericarditis were unmistakable and left no doubt about my need to call the doctor for help, but pericarditis associated with chemotherapy is *extremely* rare. However, the systemic infection was insidious, and I was unaware that something was wrong. My appetite was pretty good throughout treatment, but one evening I was unable to eat; by the next morning I was too weak to zip my jeans and began to cry for no apparent reason. At that point I thought to take my temperature, even though I didn't feel any symptoms of fever; I had a temp and was told to come right in. My white count was low, infection was diagnosed, so it was back to the hospital. For me, the lesson from this was to report *anything* that seemed out of the ordinary, even though it's kind of hard to sort this out when you feel generally sick anyway.

During treatment, I sometimes told people that this had better work because I could never do it again. I have finally begun to believe that I will never have to. But what I said was wrong. I could, and I would.

✓ Checklist

❑   Follow your daily treatment plan.

❑   Take your tape recorder to prechemotherapy visits.

❑   Choose music or meditation tapes for chemotherapy sessions.

❑   Ask about having a port (catheter) for chemotherapy delivery.

❑   Visit the dentist prior to starting chemotherapy.

❑   Pick out a wig in case you want one later.

❑   Arrange for someone who will take you to chemotherapy and stay with you afterward.

❑   Report *all* symptoms to your doctor.

chapter 10

Taking Care of Business

If you haven't done this already, put your insurance or Medicare card and hospital card in your wallet or whatever purse you always carry with you. It's a good idea to have these with you all the time anyway, but some of us, wanting to lessen the amount of stuff we carry with us, often leave these at home in a drawer. These are usually the first things you'll be asked for when you arrive at doctors' offices, labs, or hospitals for the first time.

You'll have to fill out forms everywhere you go, so before you are sitting in a waiting room review your family medical history, figure out the name, address, and phone number of at least one person outside of your spouse or partner who should be notified in an emergency, and have handy the names and phone numbers of referring doctors. Sometimes you will be asked the date of your last menstrual period—for some of us who are postmenopausal, that may be hard to remember! Ascertain the dates and the nature of any surgeries or important illnesses you may have had, and be able to tell the doctor if you have any allergies, to either foods or drugs. Make a list of every medication you take and how much of each one you take daily; this includes over-the-counter medications such as aspirin, ibuprofen, vitamins, minerals, and any "natural" supplements.

Your physician cannot treat you properly without this information—anything you ingest can have interactions with other drugs, so being ready with the information is a *must.* Taking a little time early on to have all of this information will make life in the waiting room simpler. Use our form to write down everything, then keep it with you.

Insurance

During every phase of your treatment you will be bombarded by forms from your insurance company, whether you're in an HMO, a PPO, or a pay-per-visit plan. Get out your policy and find out what will be covered and how the costs will be paid. Three common methods are used:

1. Costs are billed directly to the company, with the patient paying a co-pay at the time of service.

2. Costs are billed directly to the company, and any percentages not paid by the company will then be billed by the doctor to the patient.

3. The patient sometimes has to pay all costs up front and submit receipts to the insurance company for reimbursement.

Your company may handle your coverage in another way, so be familiar with how your particular plan works. Also, check your insurance plan to see if it covers medications. If it does, be sure to save all of the receipts, and MAKE COPIES OF THEM, before you send them off to the insurance company.

The printouts that come from insurance companies can be confusing and depressing in their complexity. Call your company and get the name of one person you can ask for any time you have a question. It helps to talk to the same person each time you need to call.

Often the paperwork is informative and helpful; however, companies sometimes make mistakes or send conflicting reports about what they have paid and what you owe. Have a large envelope or accordian-type file folder or even a box to keep

MEDICAL INFORMATION FORM

Personal Information

1. **Your name,** address, and telephone number (for when your mind isn't working well or when someone has to fill this out for you) _____

   _____

   _____

2. **Your employer's** name, address, and telephone number _____

   _____

   _____

3. **Your spouse's** name, address, and telephone number (if different from yours) _____

   _____

4. **Your spouse's employer's** name, address, and telephone number _____

   _____

   _____

Insurance Information

5. Name of company _____

   _____

6. Name of insured _____

   _____

7. Address of company and telephone number _____

   _____

   _____

8. Policy or group numbers, Social Security number of insured _____

   _____

   _____

9. Have your insurance card with you—they *always* make a photocopy.

Medical History

10. Surgeries and dates _____

    _____

    _____

    _____

11. Serious illnesses and dates (include hospitalizations) _____

_____

_____

_____

12. Prescription medications and dosages _____

_____

_____

_____

13. Nonprescription medications, including vitamins and other supplements

_____

_____

_____

14. Drug allergies _____

_____

15. Date of last menstrual period _____

_____

16. Date of last mammogram and location _____

_____

Physicians

17. Primary care physician's name, address, phone number _____

_____

18. Referring physician's name, address, phone number _____

_____

_____

19. Physician other than above you want information sent to _____

_____

_____

Other

Name, address, and phone number of someone who does not live with you to notify in case of an emergency _____

_____

_____

(relationship) _____

everything in—keep all letters and other correspondence until every bill is settled to your satisfaction.

You will probably have very little trouble with these things, but if the company's statements seem to be inaccurate and you can't get information from your insurance company, there is an agency that can help you. Most, if not all, states have a state insurance commission; its mandate is to make sure insurance companies do the right thing. If you have difficulty with a company, you can file a complaint with your state insurance commission. Also, some hospitals have a special service that helps retirees or elderly persons file for Medicare and supplemental insurance benefits.

Financial Matters

Clearly, many people face significant financial problems when they have an expensive-to-treat illness such as breast cancer. Oncology social workers should have information on Medicaid and other options. You can also talk to your city or county department of social services for advice and help. Y-ME offers a 40-page "Financial Resource Guide" containing financial options and information as well as contact information. This guide is free, and you should call Y-ME at 1-800-221-2141 to get it.

Legal Matters

Although this may seem like the last thing you need to be thinking about, there are a couple of things to go over here.

1. Will: Many of us do not have a will, sometimes because we are young and haven't thought about such things, but if you die without one, the courts will determine what happens to your property. Although you may think the courts will take care of things properly, what might make legal sense to a court would not be what you would want at all. A will takes care of this for you, because the courts must abide by what you wish. Try to do this as soon as you can. If you use an attorney, you can be confident that your will conforms to the laws of your state and actually says what you want it to. Also, an attorney can advise you what to do if you have a confusing family situation or a lot of property. If you think you can't afford an attorney, call the Legal Aid Society in your city or county.

2. Living Will: Some states and hospitals require you to have a living will. Even if they don't require it, your hospital may have a form available. This document directs your family and physicians regarding treatments you want to receive or to have withheld in case you cannot tell them yourself. This may include the following items:

- Setting forth your directions regarding medical treatment
- Expressing your right to refuse treatment and requesting care you do want
- Listing specific treatments you do not want, such as cardiac resuscitation, mechanical respiration, artificial feeding/fluids by tube
- Adding instructions for care you do want, such as pain medication or a preference to die at home if possible
- Designating someone (a proxy) to see that your wishes are carried out

  (see the sample form on page 127)

3. Power of Attorney: In a power of attorney you designate a person you trust to do business for you if you can't do it yourself. An example of what your proxy might do is pay your bills from your bank accounts. Many of us have a spouse who can do these things without a power of attorney, but others may have to rely on a family member or significant other for this. A medical power of attorney gives your proxy the legal right to direct your medical care if you can't; a living will only states your wishes. You will probably need to have a lawyer draft powers of attorney so they conform to the laws of your state.

4. Guardianship Appointment: If you have minor children who have no other parent to assume responsibility for them in case of your inability to care for them, it might be wise to appoint a guardian for them. An attorney can give you the best advice about how or whether to proceed with this document. Sometimes this appointment is included in a will.

The thought of having legal matters to tend to may be overwhelming or frightening, but taking care of them will make it easier to do the most important thing—getting well. Signing a will or a living will or a power of attorney does not mean anything about whether or not you will live or die. It just makes good sense.

Work Matters

1. Talking with Your Employer: You will need to assess the climate where you work; some people feel they need to keep their problems to themselves unless it becomes absolutely necessary to tell what is going on. You need to know, though, that it is sometimes impossible to continue to work during some kinds of treatment, so you must consider the best way to handle that. Our opinion is that openness usually works the best. However, if you think you might lose your job or that people may discriminate against you because of your illness, you should learn about your legal rights. Under the Americans with Disabilities Act, you can't lose your job simply because you have cancer if you work for an organization with 15 or more employees. To find out exactly what your employment rights are, write the National Coalition for Cancer Survivorship, 1010 Wayne Avenue, Seventh Floor, Silver Spring, MD 20910, or phone 1-301-650-8868. NCCS has several informative free publications for cancer patients.

2. Leave of Absence: Before you need it, find out how much sick leave you have and how liberal your employer will be. If you can let your employer know the situation, your employer will appreciate being able to plan for your temporary replacement if you end up having to take a leave of absence while you are in treatment. The National Coalition for Cancer Survivorship's pamphlets may help you with this problem.

3. Disability Insurance: If you are employed, even if you are self-employed, you may have some insurance that covers disability. Even though you don't stop working entirely during your treatment, you may be entitled to some disability income after a period of time. If you are, your physician will have to verify and explain your disability to the insurer. Physicians take care of these things all the time; don't feel you are imposing if you need written statements for an employer or insurance company.

Getting Help

If you live alone, or even if you don't, you will need help with some things. Here are a few things to consider:

1. Treatments: Have someone take you to and from your treatments. After a chemotherapy treatment, and sometimes later on in radiation therapy, you shouldn't drive. If you have family and friends you can depend on, this is the time to enlist their help. You need to have someone with you for the 48 hours after a chemotherapy treatment to help with your general care, meals, and especially medication schedules. If your caregivers want you to come to their house during that time, do it. You can go home as soon as you are ready, and if you have your own pillow and teddy bear it won't matter what bed you sleep in. If you have no one who can help you in this way, talk to your hospital oncology department, which should be able to suggest how to get help. The American Cancer Society's Reach to Recovery program has volunteers who give cancer patients all kinds of practical assistance. Find such a service: If this is a private company and you will be paying them, be sure they are bonded; put Grandmother's pearls in the safe deposit box; do everything you can to make it so you have nothing to worry about but getting well.

2. Household Help: If you can't afford this, ask a good friend to help you clean every couple of weeks. If you can swing hiring

LIVING WILL DECLARATION (Sample Form)

To my family, my doctors, and all those concerned with my care:

I,_____, being of sound mind, make this statement as a directive to be followed if I become unable to participate in decisions regarding my medical care.

1. If I should be in an incurable or irreversible mental or physical condition with no reasonable expectation of recovery, I direct my attending physician to withhold or withdraw treatment that merely prolongs my dying. I further direct that treatment be limited to measures to keep me comfortable and to relieve pain.

2. These directions express my legal right to refuse treatment. Therefore, I expect my family, doctors, and everyone concerned with my care to regard themselves as legally and morally bound to act in accord with my wishes, and in so doing to be free of any legal liability for having followed my directions.

3. I especially do not want: _____

_____

_____

4. Other instructions or comments: _____

_____

_____

5. Should I become unable to communicate my instructions as stated above, I designate the following person to act in my behalf:

Name: _____
Address: _____

If the person I have named above is unable to act on my behalf, I authorize the following person(s) to do so:

Name: _____
Address: _____

This Living Will Declaration expresses my personal treatment preferences. The fact that I may have also executed a document in the form recommended by state law should not be construed to limit or contradict this Living Will Declaration, which is an expression of my common-law and constitutional rights.

Signed: _____ Date: _____

Witness: _____ Witness: _____

Address: _____ Address: _____

_____ _____

Keep the signed original with your personal papers at home. Give signed copies to doctors, family, and proxy. Review your Declaration from time to time; initial and date it to show it still expresses your intent.

someone to clean for you occasionally, do it, and save the friends for your personal comfort and support. Just the basics are enough; your floor doesn't have to be clean enough to eat off of, but having things put away, laundry done, and a modicum of cleanliness is comforting. Some of us need less of this than others, but it helps to not let things pile up on you.

3. Child Care: If you have young children, you will need help with child care. Your children will need a break from the intensity and turmoil of the weeks and months of treatment. Grandparents are often wonderful for this; they may feel bewildered and uncertain about what they can do for you, and it might be just the thing for both them and your children if they can take them to their house for a weekend or pick them up for a while after school. One problem with this is that they may be too far away to help with this easily. You probably shouldn't bring them into your home for the duration unless you can let them take over for you and not regard this as a visit, causing you or your spouse more work. This you do not need. Dear friends will help with your children if you ask them—this is a task that is unrelated to all the medical stuff that goes on and is sometimes easier for someone uncomfortable dealing with that aspect of your life. Be sure that, whatever you do, you sound out your children's feelings about who they stay with and when.

❏   ❏   ❏

Earlene's Story

In the week between learning the overwhelming news that I had breast cancer and when I went in for a lumpectomy and axillary lymph node dissection, I completely closed my psychiatry practice. It was an unbelievable week. I was off balance emotionally so I contacted trusted colleagues for consultation on how I was managing this transition with my patients in the hope that the damage done to them would be minimal. These consultants made themselves available at any time for advice on how to proceed.

My colleagues came to my aid in other critically important ways. Many of them, already overworked, stepped in and agreed to see or talk with one or more of my patients while I left my practice to get well. Not one hesitated; they pitched in with love and concern.

So did my patients. Hurt and sad, many sent cards and wished me well.

My surgery was scheduled for a Saturday morning, and on Friday evening my husband and I packed up some charts and some of my plants from the office. A friend in my office building kept the rest of my plants watered and alive. I closed the office door not knowing when I would be back. It was one of the most sad and scary times in my life. I was also so angry. Within a matter of a few days, life as I had known it was over and I had to find ways to cope with this incredible challenge. Whereas I had predominantly seen myself as the caregiver, abruptly I was the patient. I had no idea at that time how very much I was to learn about being a patient.

I was away from my practice a total of ten weeks. I took enough time to complete my radiation treatments before returning to work. I am very pleased at how well I took care of myself so that when I returned to work I was sufficiently recovered to do a good job. Being self-employed, I had some disability coverage, but not at the level of my earnings, so I was worried about all the lost income. I lost interest in material goods so I wasn't concerned about spending much money other than what was required for medical treatment. I had private health insurance that allowed me to choose my doctor and hospital. The only drawback was a fairly high deductible. They were very responsive and prompt in their payments and receptive when I called with questions.

Having had breast cancer continues to be expensive. Tamoxifen costs about $100 a month, and there are the frequent checkups. My insurance paid the same benefits for medication as for other medical treatments, and I got money back for medication costs.

I became pretty reclusive during part of the treatment time. Generally, my husband did everything. He is a terrific cook, and I don't think I would have eaten had he not been there making good things.

Since radiation treatments are so much easier than chemotherapy, there was no immediate need to complete a living will. However, we decided to complete one after the treatments were over and I had more energy to deal with it.

Now I am back to work. My practice is busy and satisfying. My challenge now is to remember not to get too busy. I have to remember that exercise, good nutrition, meditation, massage, and talking with friends is not just for when I am sick. It is a new way of living.

Joann's Story

I was lucky enough to have someone who came in every other week to help clean, but my husband did everything else—laundry, cooking, shopping, taking me to treatments, being with me at the hospital, paying the bills. Looking back, I can't imagine how he did it. It is so hard for one person to take over what the other does, to support them both emotionally, and to continue to work as always.

Because I have a husband, I didn't need to give a power of attorney to anyone, and I already had made a will. When we both signed living wills, it upset the person who witnessed them for us, but we were glad to have done it. As soon as I had completed my treatments, we visited an attorney who helped us make new wills, including powers of attorney that would become effective if one of us could not make medical decisions for ourselves. I cried a lot over possibilities such as whether or not my husband would remarry if I died, who would take care of my aging mother if she survived me, whether or not my children would have any inheritance—all bridges I didn't need to cross and all resolvable. As soon as the legal work was done, I left these worries behind.

I had a really terrific work situation. My school principal was extremely supportive, as were my teammates, and as my treatment progressed and I became less able to teach, everyone helped out. When it became impossible for me to work, I stayed home to get well, and school went on. I had nearly enough sick leave for the time I needed, and the school district allowed me to borrow enough to cover the rest. If I had needed it, disability leave was an option for me. My job was waiting when I was ready to come back.

I had no problems with insurance. My medical bills were handled through a PPO. All providers billed the insurance company first, and we paid whatever was left. I was fortunate—after my expenses reached a certain level, everything was fully covered. After a separate deductible, my PPO covered 80 percent of prescription costs. Even under the best insurance coverage, cancer is still expensive.

✓ Checklist

❑   Put your insurance or Medicare card in your wallet.

❑   Contact your insurance company for the latest
      information on your coverage and the procedures to be
      followed.

❑   Make a list of information for doctors:
      Referring doctors
      Emergency phone numbers
      All medications/vitamins/over-the-counter drugs

❑   Take care of legal matters:
      Power of attorney
      Living will
      Will
      Guardian for minor children

❑   Notify your employer:
      Assess the climate of your workplace and how your
      job might be affected.
      Find out about sick leave and/or leave of absence.
      Find out about disability insurance or leaves.

❑   Arrange for help:
      Someone to accompany you to doctors' visits and/or
      treatment
      Household help
      Child care

chapter 11

The Next Five Years

After you have finished your treatments for breast cancer, you're well, aren't you? You need to be aware that the answer to that question is "No." Some doctor or another will be following you for at least the next five or ten years, probably longer. Our oncologist told us that although the chances of recurrence of breast cancer diminish with time (and there are some benchmarks: two years, five years, ten years, even fifteen), this is one of the cancers about which, at least so far, patients are not told they are "cured." This alone makes living with breast cancer especially hard, because you're never totally free of the fear that it could come back.

So how do you live with that? At first you think about it daily. It wakes you up at night. It catches you in the middle of a meal. It hits you while you are looking in the mirror. You simply can't believe how many references there are to breast cancer in the media. Every breast cancer death, whether of a personal acquaintance or of someone famous like Linda McCartney, shakes you up. You think you can never possibly forget. But the human mind is a strange and powerful thing, and as you survive the months and the years, the times when you think about having breast cancer get further and further apart, until finally it is only there when you want it to be, or when a specific event or concern brings it up again. Amazing. But it does happen.

Not surprisingly, we think we know a few more things that will help you along the way.

Be Vigilant

Being vigilant does not mean you need to obsess about what has happened to you. What it does mean is that you need to be knowledgeable about what you should watch for, and you need to be faithful about going back to your doctor for follow-up visits after your treatment has concluded. The length of time between these checkups will probably widen, and after five years you may see your oncologist only once a year. Of course, that will depend on your doctor's procedures and the kind of breast cancer or treatments you have had. Your doctor will tell you how often to have a mammogram and/or a chest X-ray. Make those appointments **and keep them.**

At your checkups you can expect to have the thorough kind of examination you had when your treatment was ongoing: The doctor will order blood tests; she will check your eyes, ears, mouth and throat; she will check lymph nodes in your neck, upper chest, underarms; she will examine your breasts, listen to your lungs and heart, feel the organs in your abdomen; she might look at your legs, feet, and hands; she will thump up and down your spine and shoulder blades, squeeze your ribs, and ask questions about your general health and stamina; she will tell you the results of chest X-rays and mammograms. She should ask you if there is anything *you* are concerned about. That is the least you should expect—she may do more.

Even though your doctor is thorough each time you have an appointment, there are things you need to do between visits. The first and most important thing is to do a breast self-examination a few days after your menstrual period each month or on the first of every month if you no longer have periods. If by now you don't know what to do, ask for instructions and follow them to the letter. Don't skip underarms. Don't wait until another day.

Anxiety and, sometimes, depression are common reactions to the conclusion of your treatment. You have been under your doctor's watchful eye for a long time, and it is hard not to have something being "done" to make you well. It is also common to be anxious during the lengthening time between checkups; you want that reassurance that you are indeed okay. These anxieties are normal. Read Wendy Harpham's excellent book, *After Cancer,* especially pages 215–260 and 266–271.

The thing to do about these anxieties is to call the doctor if you have any questions at all. You know your body better than anyone, and you know what is unusual for you. At first you will have lots of uncertainties, because many small things that never bothered you before your cancer will get your attention. Coughing for what seems a little too long? Call. The doctor may want you to have a chest X-ray, which is not much to do to get some reassurance. Feel something strange when you examine your breasts? Call. The doctors will be delighted to tell you you're feeling a rib—but let them tell you that. Whatever you do, don't spend time worrying about things. Call. Nobody will think you're being paranoid. Your body has given you reason to question it, and the best thing to do is to get your questions answered. Ask your doctor to give you a list of the kinds of problems you should call about and to describe in detail where and what kinds of things should concern you. You will begin to learn as you are watchful which pains are normal and which ones are not, and as you learn this you become easier within your body and more relaxed about living with cancer.

It is also normal to be extra-anxious around the time of your checkups. You may even not want to go for fear that your doctor will find your cancer has recurred. Try to trust your instincts; if you have followed our advice about calling the doctor with questions, about being faithful with self-exams, about not putting off anything you may find, you will already know it is likely you are all right this time. Your significant other may be even more fearful and anxious than you are, because he or she doesn't live in your body, doesn't know, deep down, the way you can, how things are.

Self-Care

Don't forget to continue your routine plans for self-care—and revise them when they grow boring. We found that the postdiagnosis self-care zeal tended to wear off, and then it was time for a change. Change your exercise program, try a new activity, buy a new relaxation tape.

In addition to your vigilance about new symptoms in general, remember to be on the watch for lymphedema.

Helping Others

There are lots of ways to help. When you are feeling well, you may want to be available to newly diagnosed women to help them through. One thing everyone can do is to encourage family and friends to do regular breast exams and to have their mammograms on schedule. Confront those who say, "I just don't have time," or "I don't have any risk factors." Tell them that more than 80 percent of women diagnosed with breast cancer don't have any risk factors. It won't prevent other women from getting cancer, but it may lead to early detection and early treatment—so important.

When you feel like it, run the "Race for the Cure." (You can walk if you don't want to run.) Buy some breast cancer postage stamps, or support other fund raisers for breast cancer research. Attend local programs for breast cancer survivors. Make new friends.

Free at Last

The last thing we want you to do is to remember daily, not just when you need them, the many ways you have been able to make

yourself feel better while you were being treated. Use them.
Read this book again. Be good to yourself. Exercise. Eat properly.
Make time for yourself and your family. Work on understanding
your place in the scheme of things. Realize, unbelievably, that
having cancer has given you a gift, one you can use over and
over for the rest of your life—a gift of renewed appreciation for
your life, for your family and friends, a gift of new and enriched
ways of living that can make all your years more fulfilled. When
you know these things, you will be free.

✔ Checklist

❏   Be vigilant.

    Do monthly breast self-exams.

    Don't skip your follow-up exams.

    Call your doctor about *any* symptoms or fears.

❏   Apply what you've learned.

    Continue taking care of yourself.

    Go over the recommendations in this book—they will
help you for your lifetime.

❏   Help someone else.

Glossary

algorithm   a step-by-step procedure for solving a problem

anesthesia   medical technique of reducing or abolishing pain to enable surgery to be performed (see *general anesthesia* and *local anesthesia*)

axillary lymph node dissection   removal of the lymph nodes in the armpit adjacent to the involved breast for microscopic examination

biopsy   removal of a small piece of tissue for microscopic examination

blood count   the numbers of different blood cells in a specified volume of blood; an important tool for diagnosis

carcinoma   cancer

chemo brain   forgetfulness or confusion that is a sometimes joked about as being a side effect of chemotherapy treatment

chemotherapy   treating disease with chemical substances

core needle biopsy   a biopsy performed with the assistance of ultrasound images or computer images using the mammogram

cradle   a framework used to hold a body part in a specific position for radiation treatment

depression   a mental state characterized by excessive sadness

dissection   cutting apart and separating body tissues

dosimetrist   someone who calculates appropriate amounts of radiation for cancer treatment

duct cells   breast cells that carry the secretions of the breast

edema   swelling

fine needle aspiration   biopsy performed by inserting a thin needle into the suspicious area and withdrawing a few cells for examination

flap reconstructive surgery   a type of reconstructive surgery that uses one's own body's tissues to create a new "breast"

general anesthesia   total unconsciousness, usually achieved by a combination of injections or gases

hormone-positive   growth of a breast cancer tumor is promoted by either estrogen or progesterone hormones

hormone therapy   treating disease with substances produced by the body, or using synthetically produced hormones such as tamoxifen

implant   a silicone envelope filled with either saline or a silicone gel to create a reconstructed breast

in situ   the cells are confined to the original duct or lobule and have not spread to surrounding breast tissue

intravenous or I.V.   injected into a vein

invasive   cancer cells have spread to surrounding breast tissue

libido   interest in sex

lobular cells   breast cells that can produce milk

local anesthesia   abolishes pain in a specific area of the body

lumpectomy   surgical removal of a breast tumor and a limited amount of associated tissue

lymph   the tissue fluid passed through a series of filters called lymph nodes

lymph node dissection   removing some lymph nodes

lymph nodes   small swellings along the lymphatic system, which bathes body tissues with fluid

lymphedema   a buildup of fluid in the arm because lymph drainage is impaired, resulting in swelling (edema)

malignant   cells that invade and destroy the tissue in which they originate and can spread to other sites in the body

mammogram   an X-ray or infrared photograph of the breast

margins   the area around the lump

mastectomy   surgical removal of a breast

medical oncologist   an internal medicine physician who has specialized in cancer treatment

metastatic   cancer has spread to other parts of the body

modified radical mastectomy   breast tissue and lymph nodes are removed, but as much of the chest muscle and nerves as possible are retained

MRI   magnetic resonance imaging—a type of scan

needle biopsy   inserting a needle into the area to remove cell material

open or **surgical biopsy**   suspicious tissue is removed through a surgical incision

pathologist   a physician who carefully analyzes samples of the breast tissue and lymph nodes and reports the nature and cause of the disease

pericarditis   an inflammation of the membrane surrounding the heart

plastic surgeon   a surgeon who specializes in correcting deformed body parts

port   a catheter that is put into a vein (often below the collarbone) and usually remains in place until the completion of all chemotherapy treatments

positive   the suspected disease is present

prostheses   artificial replacements

quadrantectomy   removal of as much as one-fourth of the breast

radiation   X-ray

radiation oncologist   a physician cancer specialist who oversees radiation treatment for cancer treatment

radiation therapy   treating disease by X-ray or radioactive substances

radical mastectomy   the breast tissue, chest muscles, and lymph nodes are all removed, as well as much of the skin, which is sometimes replaced by a skin graft

radiologist   a physician specialist who interprets X-rays to help diagnose disease

sexuality   how you feel about yourself as an attractive and sexual person

simple mastectomy   removal of breast tissue only

stage   classification of cancerous tumors based on their size and extent of spread

stereotactic biopsy   a needle is guided into the biopsy area by a computer using images from the mammogram

surgery   treating disease by operation

surgical drain   a tube inserted during surgery to prevent accumulations of fluid that may become infected or cause swelling

systemic infection   an infection of the whole body rather than individual parts

tamoxifen   a medication that blocks growth-promoting effects of estrogen on the tumor

tattoo   an indelible mark made by inserting pigment under the skin or by the production of scars

titanium dioxide or **zinc oxide**   a sun block

ultrasound   a picture made by using high-frequency sound waves

Resources and References

Alter, Michael J. (1990). *Sport Stretch*. Champaign, IL: Leisure Press. A guide to stretches for the entire body.

American Cancer Society. Pamphlets of Special Interest to Cancer Patients (free of charge). Call 1-800-ACS-2345 or the office listed in your telephone directory or write the ACS office nearest you.

Derma Sciences. Call 1-800-825-4325 for information about the Marsupial Pouch described in Chapter 7.

Food and Drug Administration's Breast Implant Information Service at 1-888-463-6332. You may have to listen to a long menu to find this information, but persist if you want the latest information on FDA regulated medical products such as breast implants.

Harpham, Wendy (1994). *After Cancer*. New York: W.W. Norton & Company, Inc., especially pages 215–260 and 266–271.

Helgeson V S, Cohen S, Schulz R, Yasko, J (1999). Education and peer discussion group interventions and adjustment to breast cancer, Archives of General Psychiatry 56:340–347.

Institute of Human Development (1986). "Tropical Ocean." Ojai, CA: Institute of Human Development. This tape contains subliminal healing messages.

Kabat-Zinn, Jon (1994). "Mindfulness Meditation in Everyday Life." New York: Sound Horizons Audio-Video, Inc. You might also be interested in a more in-depth workshop presentation called "Mindfulness Meditation Workshop: Exercises and Meditations."

Kübler-Ross, Elisabeth (1969, 1997). *On Death and Dying*. New York: Touchstone. This is the landmark book defining stages of grieving death.

Love, Susan (1995). *Dr. Susan Love's Breast Book*. Reading, MA: Addison-Wesley Publishing Company (paperback). A huge, fact-filled, thorough book about breast anatomy, physiology, and disease, this book can be overwhelming and sometimes frightening, because it contains more than most of us ever want to know about our breasts. Because it is so informative we are including it here in case you need more information than your doctor gives you. (Really, you should be able to ask your doctor about whatever you want to know. Persist until you get answers.)

MAMM: Women, Cancer, and Community. This magazine gives a lot of current information about women and cancer. It is available on newsstands or by subscription by calling 1-800-901-MAMM.

Myers, Esther (1997). *Yoga and You: Energizing and Relaxing Yoga for New and Experienced Students.* Boston: Shambala Publications. The poses are clearly explained and illustrated. The pictures show what you may strive to attain—don't try to force your body into positions for which it is not ready—that comes with time.

National Cancer Institute. *What You Need To Know About Cancer.* These pamphlets are designed to provide information about your specific kind of cancer and/or treatments. Call 1-800-4-CANCER and ask for the ones you want. They're free.

National Coalition for Cancer Survivorship has several informative free publications focusing on the rights of cancer patients. Call 1-301-650-8868, or write to them at 1010 Wayne Avenue, 7th Floor, Silver Spring, MD 29010.

Simonton, Carl (1995). "Cancer Recovery and Recurrence Prevention." Carson, CA: Hay House, Inc.

Stumm, Diana (1995). *Recovering from Breast Surgery: Exercises to Strengthen Your Body and Relieve Pain.* Alameda, CA: Hunter House, Inc.

The Alpha Book on Cancer & Living (1993). Alameda, CA: The Alpha Institute, especially pages 211–231.

The National Lymphedema Network at 1-800-541-3259, or check the web site: http://www.lymphnet.org.

Weil, Andrew (1997). "Eight Meditations for Health." New York: Tommy Boy Music.

Y-ME National Breast Cancer Organization. Call 1-800-221-2141 to find out if there is a chapter near you and to ask about their pamphlets and services. Two pamphlets we recommend are *Financial Resource Guide* and *When the Woman You Love Has Breast Cancer.*

Support

All of these organizations provide information and support for people and their families who are dealing with cancer.

American Cancer Society. Look for the local chapter in your phone book or call 1-800-ACS-2345. Available 24 hours a day, they will be able to give you information about cancer and about local patient support services. Spanish-speaking representatives are available to help you.

Susan G. Komen Breast Cancer Foundation (1-800-462-9273). If you live in a larger city there may be a chapter of this group in your town. Sometimes volunteers from this organization who have had breast cancer will call you to offer support even if you don't call them. But don't wait for them to call if you need help. Their web site is http://www.komen.org.

The Mautner Project for Lesbians with Cancer. Visit the web site: http://www.mautnerproject.org.

Y-ME National Breast Cancer Organization. This nonprofit organization with chapters in large cities provides information, referral, and emotional support to breast cancer patients and their families. Its 24-hour, 7-days-a-week national hotline number is 1-800-221-2141 (Spanish, 1-800-986-9505). Men are encouraged to call the hotline and ask to speak to a man who can help with the special concerns of partners.

Your local hospital should be able to direct you to support groups in which you can talk with others who are experiencing what you are. Some large metropolitan hospitals have a cancer center that includes a library of books and other resources that you can check out. The hospital social worker will help you deal with financial issues, transportation, and many other problems.

Internet Web Sites

The breast cancer information clearinghouse lists more than ninety web sites. We have listed above several web sites we think might be of interest to you. A good way to approach this is to use a search engine (Yahoo works very well): Search first for a broad keyword such as health, click on diseases, then cancers; keep narrowing down to breast cancer, then to other topics such as tamoxifen or nutrition, for example. Be aware that these web sites represent a huge variety of approaches to the treatment of breast cancer. You will have to sort out the ones that appeal to you. Again, we'd like to say that we believe alternative therapies should be used in conjunction with, not instead of, traditional medical care.

Index